THE WAY TO EAT

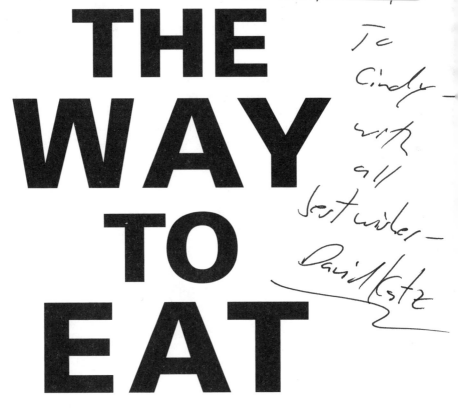

To Cindy — with all best wishes — David Katz

A Six-Step Path to Lifelong Weight Control

DAVID L. KATZ, M.D., M.P.H., F.A.C.P.M.

Yale School of Medicine

and MAURA HARRIGAN GONZÁLEZ, M.S., R.D.

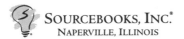

SOURCEBOOKS, INC.®
NAPERVILLE, ILLINOIS

Published by Sourcebooks, Inc.
P.O. Box 4410, Naperville, Illinois 60567-4410
(630) 961-3900
FAX: (630) 961-2168
www.sourcebooks.com

Library of Congress Cataloging-in-Publication Data

Katz, David L., MD.
  The way to eat : a six-step path to lifelong weight control / by David Katz, and Maura González.
       p. cm.
Includes bibliographical references.
  1. Nutrition—Popular works. 2. Food preferences—Popular works. 3. Nutritional anthropology—Popular works. 4. Nutritionally induced diseases—Prevention—Popular works. I. González, Maura. II. Title.
  RA784 .K327 2002
  613.2—dc21

                              2002010546

Printed and bound in the United States of America
           BG   10   9   8   7   6   5   4   3   2   1

It is the position of the American Dietetic Association that successful weight management to improve overall health for adults requires a lifelong commitment to healthful lifestyle behaviors emphasizing eating practices and daily physical activity that are sustainable and enjoyable.

We dedicate *The Way to Eat* to you, our reader. As we offer our guidance along the way to nutritional health, we honor your commitment to following it. In allying our *way* to your will, we are proud to be your partners.

Acknowledgments

The list of colleagues who have shaped our views, and in the process shaped this book, is too long for us to even know for certain where it should begin, let alone end. *The Way to Eat* traverses a landscape of knowledge and expertise in nutrition, physiology, evolutionary anthropology, dietetics, and behavior change. To the colleagues, predecessors, and mentors who discovered, explored, and charted this territory, we offer our profound appreciation, and our respect. We extend particular thanks to Dr. Linda Bartoshuk of the Yale School of Medicine, and Dr. Kelly Brownell of Yale University.

We are grateful to our publisher, Sourcebooks, and to the American Dietetic Association, in particular to Diana Faulhaber. We thank our editor, Deborah Werksman at Sourcebooks, for that artful blend of love and discipline required to move writers along from wanting to write, to having written!

While we freely acknowledge the profound contributions of so many others to this work, we must accept responsibility for any of its deficiencies ourselves. While hoping that no error, miscalculation, or misstatement has been made or will be found, we apologize in advance on the chance that despite our meticulous care, one or more will be.

We are grateful to those we love, and who love us best, for putting up with the often painful process that underlies the production of any book worth writing.

From Maura Harrigan González: To my loving husband Carlos, and my beautiful daughters, Gabriela and Ana—thank you for your constant cheerfulness and support.

From David L. Katz: I extend thanks to members of my family who lent their expertise, based on eating every day of their lives, to reading and editing *The Way to Eat*, including my mom, Susan Katz, and my sister, Liz Katz, Ph.D., who gave generously of her expertise as a clinical psychologist as well. I thank my dad, Dr. Donald Katz, a cardiologist, for sharing the very uncommon "common sense" dietary counseling he has provided to patients for the past thirty years.

My wife Catherine, my best friend, and my best editor, shows me the way, all the time. For the wonderful meals, the constructive criticism, the hours invested, and the hours surrendered, I am profoundly grateful. To Catherine, and our children—Rebecca, Corinda, Valerie, Natalia, and Gabriel—my thanks for your patience and amazing understanding, and my love beyond all measure.

Table of Contents

Introduction

Polar bears in the Sahara Desert are apt to find themselves in serious trouble. Not because of anything wrong with the bears. Rather, simply and obviously, because such bears in the Sahara would not be where they belong. Not being in the environment for which all of their remarkable adaptations prepare them places the polar bears in jeopardy.

Just like polar bears, human beings, *Homo sapiens*, are a species. And like all species, we have a native habitat and a relationship with it. We have compensated admirably for climate and terrain, using our ingenuity to devise air conditioning and heating systems, building materials, and clothes for heat and cold. But we are adapted to a particular *nutritional* environment, and in moving outside of it, we have not done so well.

This matters, and matters profoundly, for two reasons. First, a species in the wrong environment is a lot different from individuals lacking willpower. Individuals have blamed themselves for being overweight, beat themselves up for not eating right or exercising, and felt like failures for not staying on a "diet," but they have simply not understood the plight of the *species*. Polar bears are designed to retain and conserve heat. It's not their fault; it's just a fact. In the Arctic it keeps them alive. In the Sahara it would threaten their survival. We, adapted to a world where getting food was always a struggle, are designed to retain and conserve food energy (calories). In a world of subsistence, where there is barely enough, it kept us alive. In a world of constant abundance, it is threatening our well-being, and at times even our survival.

A majority of American adults are overweight. Diabetes is epidemic. Obesity causes, or contributes to, nearly four hundred thousand premature deaths annually. The chronic disease and psychological toll of an eating pattern at odds with our needs and adaptations is quite overwhelming.

The second reason this matters is that we are, as the saying goes, smarter than the average bear! And so, if we understand the specific ways in which we are designed for a world of too little food, we can apply strategies that will allow us to achieve dietary health and weight control even in a world of constant abundance.

Then & Now

The mood of a Neanderthal living one hundred thousand years ago may well have risen to optimism or sunk to despair in concert with the flesh between their ribs. In that world, the struggle to survive was simply all abiding. Living was the time spent between the fear and anxiety of an empty belly, and the calm, reassuring comfort of fullness.

Now, we all struggle against the hazards of plenty with a Stone Age physiology, and persistent Stone Age attitudes and inclinations. We are still very much what the circumstances of our evolutionary past have made us, and cannot stop being who and what we have always been just because the environment has changed, any more than polar bears, set down in the Sahara, could suddenly stop being or acting like polar bears.

The creatures we are designed to be by countless evolutionary ages and the slow, steady sculpting of natural selection cannot be denied. Our ancestors adapted to a world of intense physical labor in which getting enough food was a constant struggle. And the adaptations that resulted, that enabled their survival, have been passed along to every one of us. Just as some of us are taller, shorter, darker, lighter, faster, or slower than others, so too, do we differ with regard to our metabolism and physiology. But that variation all occurs over a range designed for surviving in a world of too little food, not too much. So, until you are prepared to blame a polar bear in the desert for overheating, you cannot blame yourself for struggling to avoid overeating, to control your weight, or to optimize your health, in the modern nutritional environment.

You can overcome the challenge of the modern nutritional environment by understanding it and our relationship with it. *Understanding and knowledge* are the basis for *power*—the power to meet challenges, to surmount barriers, to convert obstacles into opportunities. We are confronted with a modern nutritional environment that is at odds with our every trait and tendency, that is in many ways toxic to us, very much like polar bears in the Sahara. But with power born of knowledge, and with will based on realistic hope, we can get home from here. There is, indeed, a *way*.

Is This Book for You?

Probably! The struggle with food in our modern environment is nearly universal, and very few people have the resources they need to engage in it successfully.

Many books about weight control offer approaches that ignore the essential role of diet to overall health—this one does not. So it is also for you if you have concerns about, already have, or are at risk for, any chronic ailment, such as heart disease, cancer, diabetes, or arthritis. Because this book addresses how to eat well for overall health, it is also for you if you are healthy and would like to put nutrition to work in your efforts to remain that way.

Finally, this book is for you if you are willing to acknowledge that dietary pattern is important to health, pleasure, and weight control—and that, ideally, no one of these should be pursued at the cost of the others!

The Many Roads Not Taken

You and your family don't eat quite like anyone else. You have your way to eat. You may eat meat; you may not. You may like broccoli; you may not! You may have a particular ethnic dietary pattern, or not. We understand and respect the importance of these choices. So, even as we show "the" *way* to eat, we realize that there are, in fact, many parallel ways to eat. All of the ways lead toward a health-promoting eating pattern, and all are paved with the fundamentals of good nutrition. But you can certainly choose the particular path you like best, and the views you prefer.

Our intent is to provide you with the skills needed to navigate safely through the modern nutritional environment. Once you have these skills, once you know the way, you can choose how best to follow it. We act as a guide, but it's your trip, and you're in charge!

One Way, with Room for All

Fundamentally, there is only one explanation for weight gain and the development of being overweight: more calories taken in than burned. But there are many influences on, and possible explanations for, this imbalance. Calories burned depend, for example, on the rate of your metabolism when you're at rest, your physical activity level, and genetic influences both known, and as yet unknown, to name a few.

In our view, the best explanation for being overweight is that we are creatures designed to be metabolically efficient, living in a world where food is enticing and abundant, and physical activity often avoidable. We respect that others may have different theories, but we believe this one captures most of the important issues.

We also respect that there are many approaches to weight control and weight loss. We, however, believe that a way of eating consistent with long-term health and regular physical activity is the best means to long-term weight control.

Finally, we think that monitoring weight can be useful, but should not be a preoccupation, let alone the obsession it so often becomes. You cannot choose what to weigh. You can choose how to eat and how physically active to be. In our view, we should all focus on the things we can control. Work on a healthful lifestyle, and let weight take care of itself. The *way to eat* is a route toward healthful eating and weight control. It is moving along that route in the right direction that is the emphasis, rather than how far you choose to go.

What Is, and Is Not, Meant by "Diet"

In a book about nutrition and health, it's quite hard not to use the word "diet." So we do use it. *The Way to Eat* is about a dietary pattern, or eating habits, that is appropriate for a lifetime of good health. When we refer to "your diet," or "a diet," we generally mean your pattern of eating—the foods you choose on a day-to-day basis over time.

What we do not mean is the kind of diet associated with "dieting," the "I'm on a diet," or, "I'm off my diet," kind of diet. Except under special circumstances, we do not support "dieting," or the "on-again, off-again" kind of diet. The pattern of eating that is best suited to promote your health and control your weight is the pattern of eating you should stick with forever. This, too, is a "diet." When we use the term, we try to be very clear about exactly what we mean. But if there is ever any doubt in your mind, you can assume that we mean your usual way of eating, not a short-term effort to fit into a smaller bathing suit in time for a summer vacation!

Your Will, This Way

Food once was simple. Success, status, security, and survival itself were all represented by a full belly and a reliable supply of food.

In the modern world, however, where we have more than we need, our relationship with food has become complicated. Naturally, we still get great pleasure from eating, and a sense of security from abundance. Food may be the most readily, consistently available means of pleasure and gratification in our lives. So food is our friend, perhaps even a passion. Yet as we struggle with our waistlines, our cholesterol, our blood pressure, or blood sugar food becomes pretty frustrating, and can at times seem the cause of some serious troubles.

And yet we must reconcile. Because food is fundamental. We cannot just say "no" and turn our backs. We must eat, today, and every day after this one. Is it possible to eat and truly enjoy eating? To enjoy eating, and yet not be harmed by doing so? It is.

But you need to know *how*. And that is what makes this book different. It will tell you.

As this book will make very clear, the knowledge and skills, the metabolism and cravings, and the insights and inclinations for eating well in a world of *too little food* are indeed innate after four million years of natural selection. But in a new and unprecedented world of plenty, we must learn the needed skills to eat well, control our weight, preserve our health, and live in harmony with food. In this effort, as in most, knowledge is power.

We know *what* we should eat. You don't really doubt that fruit and vegetables are good for you, do you? Nutrition experts are nearly unanimous about a health-promoting eating pattern, and that consensus is none too different from what our mothers told us, and their mothers told them. While we may have a very clear sense of *what* we should be eating, most of us have virtually no idea *how*. There are important, fundamental influences on our food preferences that must be known to be understood, and understood to be mastered. You cannot eat a healthful diet just because you would like to, nor because you think you should, and certainly not because someone tells you to! You must know *how*. We tell you.

There is, indeed, a way to eat well for weight control, and for health, while preserving the pleasure that eating should provide. At first, it appears to be a way strewn with obstacles: primitive, long-forgotten traits; metabolic tendencies; social conventions; and cultural pitfalls. But we believe every obstacle to eating well is an opportunity for doing so waiting to be created. How do you convert obstacles to opportunities? You understand them, and you respond to them with suitable strategies. *The Way to Eat* leads to that understanding, and provides those strategies.

The Way Ahead

Your prior attempts to eat well were excursions on an unmarked trail into innumerable hazards with no map, no compass, and no guide. This book guides you on the *way to eat* well for the rest of your life in six steps. In Section I, Step 1, Knowledge, you learn why we eat as we do; why we are so much like polar bears in the Sahara; what eating pattern, or range of patterns, is suited to our health; and gain a clear understanding of what you actually are eating now.

But knowledge is not enough: it must be well applied. The application of knowledge is Power, and this is what you acquire in Section 2, Step 2, by learning the basics of behavior change. Eating is a well-established behavior, one you practice every day; changing it is not a trivial undertaking. But you can change behavior, and there is a science to guide and empower you.

Then comes Section III, four key steps along the *way* to a lifetime of health, weight control, and contentment with food. In this section, you are guided through the many potential "obstacles" to eating well in the modern world, and shown how each can be turned into an opportunity by using key skills and strategies. It is here that the *way to eat* well for the rest of your life opens up before you as you layer skill upon skill, strategy upon strategy, until you can bound right over every obstacle. In Step 3, you learn to master your metabolism. In Step 4, you learn to make use of good information and avoid bad. In Step 5, you learn to resist and control the interactions between food and mood, the reasons we eat other than hunger. And in Step 6, as you tie together your now impressive set of skills, you learn to navigate safely through the nutritional environment.

Finally, Section IV provides the detailed resources you need to use your skills and strategies in the places, and with the people, that matter: the supermarket, cafeteria, restaurant, home kitchen, and workplace with friends, family, coworkers, and children. Offering the very paving stones of the *way to eat*, Section IV provides meal plans, recipe tips, shopping guides and cooking techniques, food label interpretation and recommended brands, what to cook, what to shop for, what to snack on, what to feed kids, what to keep in your pantry, what to order when eating out, and much more.

This is what you'll find as you set off along the way. You will learn unsuspected things about yourself, our species, and the modern nutritional environment. You will learn about obstacles to eating well you didn't even know were there, but which you probably have stumbled over nonetheless. You will learn how to convert these obstacles into opportunities. You will become knowledgeable, skillful, and resourceful. You will learn to master the modern nutritional environment, so that even if it's a desert out there, your diet is an oasis.

How will you know you are truly on your *way*, and how will the *way* change you?

- Eating well will just come naturally to you.
- You will be able to evaluate your diet honestly and accurately.
- You will be highly motivated to eat well.
- You will be satisfied with your weight, and with your ability to control it.
- You will get pleasure from eating, and from the ways your dietary pattern is affecting your health and appearance.

- You will have a healthy relationship with food, so it is not a constant preoccupation.
- You will have eating habits that promote your health, rather than threaten it.
- You will have established a healthful pattern of eating that you can live with comfortably for the rest of your life.
- You will have good self-esteem.
- You will know how to make your home a "safe" nutritional environment, in which all choices are good choices.
- You will know how to avoid overeating, or bingeing.
- You will know how to choose healthful foods wherever you go.
- You will know how to help others eat well, and to get them to help you.
- You will know how to interpret food labels.
- You will know how to select the most nutritious foods in every category at the market or grocery store.
- You will know how to snack so that you can eat whenever you get hungry, without overeating or gaining undesired weight.
- You will know how to stock a healthful pantry.
- You will know how to substitute ingredients so you can eat favorite dishes and improve their nutrition.
- You will know the most healthful ways to cook and bake.
- You will know the most nutritious brands and products in many food categories.
- You will know the obstacles to eating well, and strategies for overcoming them.
- You will know what eating pattern is appropriate to promote health, prevent disease, and control weight.
- You will understand that difficulty with eating well, or controlling weight, is not your fault.

Section One:

Knowledge

Why don't eating well, good health, and weight control just come naturally to us all? The answer resides in our one hundred thousand–year-old genes. In your efforts to eat well and control your weight, you have been tripping over the traits and tendencies of your prehistoric ancestors! Knowing this, and knowing what the obstacles to eating well are, is essential in charting a course around them!

You also need to know what diet is appropriate for health, weight control, and the enjoyment we all expect eating to provide. There is an answer, and you will learn it—or reaffirm it—here.

And finally, to get where you are going, you must also know where you are starting. To know how best to improve your diet in support of your goals for health, contentment, and weight control, you must assess your current eating habits accurately so you can tell what ought to be changed. Getting at the truth, the whole truth, and nothing but the truth about your actual dietary pattern is more challenging and subtle than you realize!

Step I:

Reconsider Yourself

(the Plight of Polar Bears in the Sahara)

PRONGHORN ANTELOPE THAT race across the plains of Colorado and Wyoming can run up to forty miles per hour, and sustain their top speed for more than four miles, even though no existing predator can come close to catching them. Why?

The presumed explanation is that thousands of years ago such predators—long-legged wolves and a North American hyena—did exist. The speed and endurance of the pronghorn developed, the way traits do in nature, as a product of natural selection. Only the antelope that escaped these predators survived to produce more antelope, and so on. The end products of this process are the traits that now define being a pronghorn antelope. And these traits cannot be changed just because they no longer happen to be necessary. The pronghorn continue to run fast and far, even though their predators are extinct; they are, in essence, running from ghosts. They share the genetic makeup of their ancestors, and thus remain what their past required them to be. And so do we.

Like other species, ours, *Homo sapiens*, lives in the modern world with prehistoric genes, and prehistoric tendencies. The human genome, the overall pattern of our genes and the blueprint responsible for much of what we are, has not changed appreciably in one hundred thousand years. Our distant ancestors' genes are our genes; therefore, their traits, their metabolism, and their physiology are ours, too.

Efforts to improve your diet initiated without considering the fundamental adaptations of our species may have led you to believe that if you "fail" to follow dietary guidelines, to "eat right," or control your weight, you have failed. It is not so.

For most species, the environments, habitats, and diets they can and cannot tolerate are on display in their physical features: the length of a coat, the presence of gills, the shape of a beak. But even though our limits are less visible than those of other species, they are no less real, and no less important. We are well suited for a particular environment, and ill suited for others. In particular, we are adapted to the *nutritional environment* of our ancestors.

The Long & Winding Road, From Then (Them) to Now (Us)

Human and prehuman history, and consequently the origins of our dietary behavior, can be traced back reliably nearly four million years. The available evidence indicates that our earliest identifiable ancestors lived primarily in trees, and were mostly, if not exclusively, plant eaters. Over hundreds of thousands of years, prehuman primates increased in size and descended from the trees. As the brain grew larger and intellect increased, our ancestors came together in cooperative groups, began to use first bone and then stone implements, and were able to scavenge successfully; this occurred several million years ago.

Our ancestors next became successful hunters in the time of *Homo erectus*, and continued to refine their skills thereafter. Hunting is thought to have become particularly important during the earliest days of our own species, *sapiens*, in particular *Homo sapiens neanderthalensis*, the so-called Neanderthals. The earliest *Homo sapiens* date back up to three hundred thousand years; Neanderthals date back approximately one hundred thousand years; Cro-Magnon man dates back up to fifty thousand years; and modern *Homo sapiens* date back approximately thirty thousand years. Thus, our genes today take us back to the Neanderthals, and before, with little change since. The saying is, "You are what you eat." But, in fact, we are what the Neanderthals ate! So, what does that mean? To understand our "native" dietary habitat, we need to understand the diet and related behavior of our great-great-great-great…grandparents. Grandmother and grandfather Neanderthal.

Gathering & Hunting, Rather than Hunting & Gathering

Our ancestors were good hunters. Even so, they apparently rarely obtained more than 30 percent or so of total calories from hunting, with the remainder obtained through gathering. Most importantly, despite the contributions of both hunting and gathering, the human food supply was always uncertain. A large kill or profusion of plants in good weather might supply plenty of food for a brief period, but this was invariably followed by periods of famine. A pattern of feast followed by famine was among the prominent characteristics of the nutritional environment to which our ancestors adapted.

This is critical: our native dietary habitat is one of persistent near-famine, interrupted by an occasional feast. We are adapted to such an environment, and that explains a lot!

For one thing, it makes very good sense that we tend to eat a lot…simply because we can! That's exactly what our ancestors must have done, and it was a good thing. A pattern of eating more than they immediately needed, and storing fat to endure periods of relative deprivation, has been observed in modern hunter-gatherers, and is thought likely to have characterized our Stone Age ancestors as well.

The same, of course, is noticeable in species other than our own. Recall, for example, watching any nature program about predators such as lions. Lean before a kill, afterward, their bellies drag all the way to the ground. Such gorging makes sense when the next meal is uncertain.

As hunter-gatherers, our ancestors of course ate meat. This suggests that we should be well adapted to eating meat too, and that doing so should not be bad for health. Yet you have doubtless heard that meat is high in saturated fat, and may contribute to the risk of heart disease and cancer. Why would the descendants of Stone Age hunters be adversely affected by eating meat? In part because meat is not what it once was.

The Urge to Splurge: Same As It Ever Was...

Ellen, age forty-one, has always struggled to control her weight. Because she doesn't trust her ability to eat in moderation, she instead avoids food altogether for as long as she can. This works pretty well during the workday, when she is busy and distracted. But by the end of the day, Ellen is starving! As a result, she eats more calories in a big dinner than she should have eaten spread out over the day, and never loses the weight she has been trying so long to lose. Frustration about the weight just keeps the pattern going, and going.

From our earliest origins, we have been designed to binge eat! Our ancestors did this because they had no choice; sometimes they had plenty of food, sometimes they had none. So when they could eat, they did. Binge eating is no longer helpful to those of us who have access to food all of the time. But the tendency is perfectly natural.

They Don't Make Meat Like They Used To
Our ancestors did not eat the kind of meat many of us do today. Modern beef cattle, for example, contain 25–30 percent fat by weight. The average fat content of free-living African antelope and other animals like them, thought to be representative of the animals our ancestors hunted, is generally under 4 percent. So in our "domestic" food animals, we have increased the fat content of meat nearly ten times! The differences go beyond the quantity of fat, to the type of fat. Modern meat is rich in saturated fat, the kind associated with raising cholesterol and increasing heart disease risk. In contrast, the flesh of wild animals is low in saturated fat, and relatively high in polyunsaturated fat, a class of fat not associated with heart disease risk. The flesh of wild game contains more than five times more polyunsaturated fat ("good" fat) per gram than is found in modern meat, and also contains omega-3 fatty acids, almost completely absent in domestic beef. You have probably heard of omega-3 fatty acids as "fish oil." It would hardly make sense for us to get benefit from a nutrient we weren't adapted to eat, and many of our ancestors, particularly those far from the coasts, ate little fish. The apparent paradox of needing

a nutrient from fish without having adapted to eat fish *per se* is resolved by knowing that only in modern times is "fish oil" limited to fish! Domestication has removed omega-3s from the flesh of animals by changing their food supply. The same thing is now happening to fish, by the way. Farm-raised salmon do not eat the algae from which their omega-3 fatty acids are produced, and are potentially becoming deficient in this nutrient class as well! We may be headed toward "domestic" fish without fish oil, just as we removed the same oil from the flesh of other animals when we domesticated them.

Back & Forth

Stone Age humans consumed far more fiber than we do, more calcium, a sixth of the current U.S. intake of sodium, and abundant vitamins due to the variety of plant foods they consumed. They generally ate much less fat than we do, although this was variable by time and place, and they may have even exceeded our intake of cholesterol, due to consumption of meat, eggs, organs, and bone marrow. Over the course of recent decades, as those of us living in modern societies have progressively consumed more fat, more sugar, more salt, less grains, and less fiber, we have moved further and further from our native diet.

Evolution of…the Couch!

Not only has the quantity and character of our food changed, but so has the way we put, or rather don't put, those calories to use. We are all subject to a truly dramatic decline in energy expenditure in modern times, and consequently a comparable decline in our need for fuel, or calories. Our ancestors were consistently lean not only because of the number of calories they ate, but because of those they burned. The same modern environment that gives us a constant, abundant food supply unlike any other in history, also gives us the technology that does the work our muscles used to do. Because technology helps make more technology, the trend toward less and less physical work is continuing and accelerating. Data in Great Britain, for example, reveal a 65 percent decline in the calories burned up in work-related physical activity since the 1950s. Over this same time period, the number of calories available to each of us has increased significantly. That combination is an obvious problem.

Sowing Civilization

While the origins of human civilization are subject to debate, most experts look to Mesopotamia, where agriculture developed in the delta of the Tigris and Euphrates rivers in what is now Iraq approximately twelve thousand years ago. The establishment of a reliable food supply for the first time in history gave rise to unprecedented population density. Repeated cycles of irrigation caused salt to precipitate in the soil, destroying its fertility. For the first time, the nutritional needs of a human population exceeded the potential yield from hunting and gathering. The large, concentrated population that agriculture had sustained was compelled to spread out in search of adequate food. As a result, civilized humans started to spread out over the planet.

Wandering Taste Buds

As early peoples left their native lands to make new lives for themselves elsewhere, they needed to adjust to variations in the environment. Each new excursion led to new climates, new soil, new plants, and resulted in the failure of certain established crops, and the successful cultivation of new ones. So, while our dietary traits and tendencies and preferences can all be traced back to our common ancestors, necessity made our ancestors flexible. We can guess that when our ancestors could not grow or find the food they loved, they learned to love what they could find or grow!

Millet and rice grew well in the Far East, so these replaced wheat and barley. Corn grew well in the Americas, and so became a staple there. The result of our species settling the entire planet was a great deal of variety in the diets of different countries and cultures. This variety is important for what it reveals about us, and for what it conceals. It reveals how importantly our tastes and food preferences are influenced by familiarity; we like what we're used to. This is important because it tells us we can be adaptable about diet, and that our taste buds are not programmed for nothing but steak and potatoes. We are all the product of common ancestors, and our basic adaptations to diet are shared among us all. We all like sugar, salt, and fat when these are made available. We all tend to eat too much when we can. We all tend to gain weight when there is enough good food available to allow us to do so.

We are, despite the wide range of cuisines around the world, much more alike than different in our basic dietary traits and tendencies. The Far East provides a clear example of this. Asian and Western diets have traditionally been very different. But as the Japanese or Chinese become more affluent, and gain access to food rich in fat, sugar, salt, and calories, these foods are as popular there as they are in the U.S.! The obesity epidemic is taking hold there as well. We're all in this together.

In trying to choose fruits and vegetables over chocolate and cheese you are fighting your own metabolism, engineered to preserve you through periods of prehistoric famine. You have been struggling with your diet, and losing, through no fault of your own; you have been running into obstacles you didn't know were there. You have been tripping over your ancestors' survival skills!

Back to Your Nutritional Future

So, reconsider yourself. Consider yourself in the light of some Ice Age dawn, the early morning mists of a primeval scene. Consider yourself not only as a person and an individual, but also as a creature, one member of a species. And as you do, forgive yourself for every thought you've ever had about too little willpower, or weakness. As you get ready to take control of your dietary health, come to terms with why you didn't have control in the first place. Our ancestors did not possess a self-discipline we lack. They simply lacked the food supply and modern conveniences we possess!

How does this help? If you know you are not at fault for your dietary struggles, you won't feel quite as burdened by them. You can begin to look at our common "food fight" as a challenge, not as a character flaw. Forgiving yourself for previous "failures" is the first key step along the actual *way to eat* well!

The Obstacle Course

The traits endowed to our ancestors, and therefore to us, by the demands of their nutritional environment make up a discrete list of challenges we face in our efforts to eat well. Our metabolism, the basic functioning of our bodies, is designed for a Stone Age environment. As a result, we like sugar, salt, and fat just as much now that they are abundantly available to us as our ancestors did when finding them was a struggle. We tend to binge, or overeat, because eating everything available made sense in the past. The center in our brains that regulates appetite is actually designed to encourage more eating when we have a variety of foods and flavors rather than just one. This may have helped our ancestors survive, but it too encourages us to overeat.

Each of these traits represents either an obstacle to eating well, or an opportunity for doing so. The difference between *obstacle* and *opportunity* is understanding. You have almost certainly been crashing into many of our prehistoric traits in your previous efforts to improve your diet or control your weight. This time will be different because you know they're there. This time, your way will lead you around, over, and past the obstacles you crashed into before.

Define Your Destination

AMONG PUBLIC HEALTH experts, there is ever-increasing appreciation for just how great an impact on health eating habits actually have. In the United States, the combination of poor diet and physical inactivity has been identified as the second leading cause of premature death, behind smoking. Partly because smoking rates are going down, but also in part because our dietary struggles seem to be worsening, current data suggest that diet and lack of activity will soon be, if they are not already, the No. 1 killers in the United States! Obesity alone accounts for an incredible one thousand preventable deaths in the U.S. *every* day!

Leave Your Doubts along the Wayside

Every ten years, the United States Department of Health and Human Services spells out health goals for the nation in the *Healthy People* guidelines. Used by policy makers, researchers, and the government, the *Healthy People* documents are almost like a bible to public health professionals. So great is the confidence among experts in what we know about diet and health that many of the *Healthy People 2010* objectives, like the *Healthy People 2000* objectives before them, relate to healthful eating. Want the punch line right away? Fruits, vegetables, and whole grains really are good for you!

There is no concise way to summarize the evidence supporting a healthful eating pattern, because it is simply too vast. The body of

Nutrition 101

What we eat falls mainly into three main macronutrient classes: protein, fat, and carbohydrate.

Carbohydrate

Carbohydrate is the primary energy source for our bodies. It comes in many varieties, from simple to complex, all of which provide four calories per gram. Sources of complex carbohydrate provide dietary fiber, the indigestible part of plants. A high intake of dietary fiber has numerous health benefits and is the cornerstone of *The Way to Eat*.

Fat

Dietary fat is an essential component of cells and hormones. However, since fat is the most concentrated source of calories, providing nine calories per gram, the amount of fat eaten should be carefully controlled.

Fats are made up of different types of fatty acids that are named for their chemical structure. While all types of fat contain the same amount of calories, their effect on health varies:

Monounsaturated fat, abundant in the Mediterranean Diet, is generally considered health-promoting. Many of the fats recommended in *The Way to Eat* are monounsaturated.

Polyunsaturated fat is generally considered health promoting, or at least harmless, depending on the variety. Some polyunsaturated fats are called essential fatty acids because they are needed in body tissues but cannot be made by the body. The two classes of essential fatty acids are omega-6 and omega-3. In particular, the omega-3 fatty acids, often called "fish oils," are considered health promoting. Omega-3 fatty acids are included in *The Way to Eat*.

Saturated and *trans fats*, found in animal products and processed food, raise cholesterol and are associated with increased risk of chronic disease. These fats are strictly limited in *The Way to Eat*.

Protein

Protein is necessary for the building, maintenance, and repair of the body's tissues. Protein comes from both animal and plant sources.

Much of the protein in *The Way to Eat* comes from plant sources since these are lower in saturated fat and higher in fiber than animal sources. An excessive protein intake is potentially harmful to the kidneys and the skeleton. The amount of protein in *The Way to Eat* is plenty to meet the body's protein needs.

Vitamins and Minerals

Collectively, vitamins, minerals, and related nutrients are referred to as *micronutrients*, because they are eaten in microscopic quantities.

Vitamins are organic compounds that are essential for health, or even survival. They have letter names that represent the sequence in which they were discovered. They are grouped into fat-soluble, or water-soluble classes. To obtain all of the vitamins needed for good health, a varied diet is required.

Minerals are inorganic compounds, generally elements, that function in human metabolism, and are essential for health. Some are needed in relatively large quantities, such as calcium, and others in very tiny amounts, such as vanadium, or tin.

evidence supporting a diet rich in grains, vegetables, and fruit, moderate in protein and in total fat, balanced in fat type, abundant in vitamins and minerals and fiber is, quite simply, overwhelming. It is based on literally thousands, tens of thousands, and perhaps even hundreds of thousands of scientific studies and papers, and on countless observations of the links between eating and health.

Confusion Is a State of Mind

You probably know that the best time to sell umbrellas, and the worst time to buy them, is when it's pouring rain. And the best time to "sell" diets is when people keep getting heavier and heavier, and more and more frustrated. But when you're frustrated and desperate for something is not the best time to be "buying" advice—because almost anything will sound good! But that's us, the population of the United States and other industrialized countries. We have been struggling with our diets, and our weight, and are pretty darned frustrated. You could sell us just about anything...and people do.

Numerous authors with varying credentials (or no credentials) offer nutrition miracles to suit any taste. High-fat diets, high-protein diets, sugar-free diets, and others promise to let us have our proverbial cake and eat it too—indulging in favorite foods, losing weight, achieving peak performance.

And, as if these distractions were not enough to generate confusion, a multi-billion dollar industry bombards us with promises about devices, lotions, potions, programs, and pills that will let us weigh whatever we want, trim our thighs, and tone our buns, without even worrying about diet! Who wouldn't sign up for that?!

Fad Diets Are Bologna (Figuratively, and Often Literally)

Why not try the many fad diets being offered today? For one very good reason: they're a bunch of bunk! In the past, the proverbial snake oil came in the form of "Dr. Fixit's Magic Cure-All Potion!" sold off a horse and buggy that didn't stay in one place long enough for Dr. Fixit to get what he deserved! Today, it's packaged in the form of fad diets.

Should you try a diet with no carbohydrate, high in protein, or high in fat? Do you need to combine foods in a highly structured way to control your weight? Have the authors of the ever-growing supply of "diet books" discovered truths that all of the "conventional" experts and professional organizations in nutrition have somehow overlooked?

No! The authors of fad diet books are simply taking advantage of the fact that following a good diet in the modern environment has proved very challenging. If we know how to adopt a health-promoting diet, the temptation of looking elsewhere, of tuning in to every fad that comes along, fades away. Combining the knowledge of "how" to eat well, with a clear understanding of "what" dietary pattern (or narrow range of patterns) promotes health is the way. Fad diets lead nowhere you want to go.

Fad Diet Fantasies & Facts

Fantasy: Popular diets produce rapid weight loss.

Fact: Much of the weight lost quickly on high-fat or high-protein

On Again, Off Again

At 5'6", and weighing just over 280 pounds, Wendy, age thirty-three, was pretty much obsessed with her weight. She had tried every diet she could find. On some of them she did lose weight. In fact, on one very restricted diet, she lost over fifty pounds, and in a relatively short period of time. But the "diet" Wendy was on was not one she could live with, so she went off—and gained back all the weight she had lost, and then some.

Until recently, when we met, Wendy was simply waiting, hopefully, for the next diet to come along. Even though such diets had failed her every time, they were the best option she could find. She now has a better option. She knows that for permanent control of her weight, she needs a lifelong way of eating, not a short-term diet. She's definitely headed the right way now.

diets is body water. This "weight" loss is neither healthy, nor sustainable. The dehydration is slowly corrected, and the weight is regained.

Fantasy: Popular diets produce weight loss and improve health by changing the distribution of carbohydrate, fat, and protein rather than by restricting calories.

Fact: All popular diets that result in short-term weight loss do so by restricting calories. The changes in macronutrient levels the diets do talk about conceals the calorie restriction that the diets don't talk about. It is the calorie restriction that causes weight loss.

Fantasy: Fad diets offer a quick fix to the chronic problem of weight control.

Fact: Fad diets are an example of the adage, "There's never time to do it right, but there's always time to do it over…and over…and over." There is no truly "quick fix" to dietary health and weight control; it takes a lifetime of eating well and being physically active to support these goals. The sooner you start down that path, the sooner you'll begin to see lasting benefit.

Fantasy: Fad diets increase energy levels.

Fact: There are testimonials that suggest a short-term boost in energy on some of the popular diets. This doesn't last long, and is not necessarily a good thing. Use of stimulant drugs also causes a short-term boost in energy, but at the cost of health, the same cost exacted by a poor diet. Not everything that makes us briefly feel good is a good idea!

Fantasy: Popular diets allow you to eat "whatever you want" and still lose weight.

Fact: Most popular diets severely restrict food choices. This, and calorie restriction, leads to short-term weight loss. You may be able to eat ice cream or sausage on a popular diet—but if you can't eat anything else, these foods lose their appeal pretty quickly. For this reason, hardly anyone stays on the popular fad diets for any length of time. That's the part the testimonials don't tell you!

Fantasy: If you lose weight or lower your cholesterol on a popular diet, you are improving your health.

Fact: Many very bad health conditions are associated with weight loss, low blood cholesterol, or low blood glucose. Good health is much more than just these measures. Fad diets do not promote health.

Fantasy: Eating carbohydrates causes weight gain by raising insulin levels. Restricting carbohydrate intake leads to weight loss, because high levels of insulin cause weight gain.

Fact: Not all carbohydrate is created equal! Complex carbohydrate foods, such as whole grains, are rich in fiber, and in fact lower blood insulin levels; this is quite different from the simple carbohydrates found in highly processed foods that tend to provide little fiber. Limiting intake of highly processed foods makes good sense for many reasons. Restricting intake of complex carbohydrates does not, and is in fact likely to be harmful. Further, insulin is involved in our use of fat and protein, as well as carbohydrate. Eating too many calories from any source leads to weight gain and higher insulin levels.

Not All Loss Is Gain

Fad diets, because they are energy restricted, do produce loss of fat as well as water. But neither loss tends to last. Water weight is regained as soon as the "diet" ends, or even before, and there is no evidence that fat loss achieved on a fad diet is sustainable. The National Weight Control

Registry, developed at the University of Colorado School of Medicine by Dr. James Hill and colleagues, compiles the best information available about strategies associated with long-term maintenance of weight loss. Care to guess what diet people successful at maintaining weight loss tend to eat? A dietary pattern very similar to that recommended by virtually all nutrition experts, and the one we contend is the *way to eat*, with most calories in the form of complex carbohydrates, less than 30 percent of calories from fat, and about 20 percent of calories from protein. Data in the Registry also highlight the importance of consistent physical activity for maintaining weight loss, another consistent recommendation among experts.

Insulin 101

Insulin has two primary functions: making fuel available immediately to cells, and storing it. When energy production is needed immediately, glucose enters cells chaperoned by insulin. Often, however, food energy exceeds the immediate need for fuel. The excess is stored for later use. A mechanism for storing food energy was of course essential to the survival of our ancestors, who at times had plenty of food, but more often faced extended periods of deprivation. The ability to fill an energy reserve in times of plenty provided the needed defense against times of want.

Most of the popular fad diets build their pitches around insulin metabolism. Sounding impressive, these arguments are generally based on a whole lot of nonsense.

Of Famine & Fat: Energy Reserves for Rainy Days

When food was relatively scarce, it is likely that a brisk release of insulin whenever food was eaten was advantageous. Acting like a sponge to sop up available food energy, insulin would result in some food energy being burned, and the excess being stored as carbohydrate (glycogen) or fat. The more vigorous the release of insulin, the more effectively every available calorie from any source—carbohydrate, fat, or protein—would be sopped up and put to use. So, prehistoric humans with a very robust insulin response were much more likely to survive than those who were less metabolically efficient.

Bad Time for a Good Tendency

Despite our ancestors' tendency to release insulin briskly and use fuel efficiently, they were never "fortunate" enough to become fat. But transplant that same mechanism to the modern world. We have access to plenty of food all of the time. A brisk release of insulin, in response to calories from any source, results in the storage of excess food energy as fat. Instead of that fat being burned for fuel, it just keeps accumulating, because every day and every meal increases the total sum of excess food energy available to us.

And then our troubles begin. Body fat, or adipose tissue, also is dependent on the actions of insulin. The more body fat there is, the more insulin is needed. Now, the tendency to release insulin briskly that led to weight gain in the first place is made worse by the weight that was gained! As demands for insulin get abnormally high, the insulin receptor starts to malfunction, leading to the state known as "insulin resistance." The conditions of our modern nutritional environment have converted what was once a beneficial state into an adverse state. This is the plight of polar bears in the Sahara!

The Way to Eat

Everything known about nutrition and health *and* insulin metabolism, indicates that a diet based predominantly on plant foods, including vegetables, grains, and fruits, moderate in total fat and balanced in type of fat, and moderate in protein intake is the very best way to lose weight and control weight over time. What good fortune that this same diet is associated with improved overall health, enhanced immune function, reduced risk of cancer, the prevention of diabetes, increased survival, and innumerable other health benefits! Contrast this to fad diets that ask you to throw out everything known about nutritional health for short-term, unsustainable weight loss.

On the basis of all of the above considerations, we recommend an eating pattern made up mostly of whole grains, vegetables, and fruits. Nuts, seeds, fish or seafood, and the right oils are also important to ensure a balance in the types of dietary fat. With regard to the major food categories, or macronutrients, our recommendations are as follows: approximately 20–25 percent of total calories from fat; approximately

60 percent of calories from mostly complex carbohydrates; and the remaining 15–20 percent of calories from protein. This pattern is based on the recommendations of all of the leading nutrition organizations in the U.S., with some consideration of our ancestral eating habits. All of the details you need to convert these recommendations into specific food choices, meals, and your way of eating are provided in Section IV.

Food Category	Recommended Intake as Percent of Total Calories
Carbohydrate	**55%–60%** *should be mostly complex*
Fat	**20%–25%** *balanced distribution of poly-unsaturated and monounsaturated fats, restricted intake of saturated and trans fats*
Protein	**15%–20%**
Fiber	A generous intake of fiber (at least 25 grams per day) is recommended. Fiber is the indigestible component of plant foods, and comes in two basic forms—soluble and insoluble—both of which offer distinct health benefits.

Get Your Bearings

OVER THE YEARS, many of our patients have told us that they "barely eat anything," and yet they still gain weight. People do have different metabolic rates, and some do gain weight on relatively few calories. However, most of us tend to underestimate the calories we take in, and overestimate the calories we are burning, or both.

Watch Out for Pitfalls
There are a variety of pitfalls to getting a realistic assessment of your diet, and if you are subject to any or all of these, they must be addressed before you set out toward a healthier way of eating.

Wishful Thinking
Eating well in the modern nutritional environment can be quite challenging. As a result, you may be tempted to *assume* you are meeting that challenge fully and successfully, when in fact you are not. This wishful thinking may lead to underestimates of fat and calorie intake, overestimates of fruit and vegetable intake, and so on.

Food Generalization
We tend to believe that the name of a food will reliably reflect its nutritional properties, but there are considerable variations within any food category. A "turkey sandwich," or "salad," or almost any other "name"

That Which We Call a Bagel...

Jeanine, thirty-one, couldn't understand why she wasn't losing weight. In particular, she noted that she ate nothing for breakfast but a "bagel." Just a bagel.

But what a bagel! What she was eating was an "everything" bagel, with a variety of seeds, nuts, and cheese, along with a generous layer of cream cheese. This particular bagel was providing nearly six hundred calories, more than three times as many as a standard bagel without spread.

What's in a "name"? Perhaps not much when talking about roses. But when talking about bagels, about four hundred calories!

---

can really represent a whole category of foods or dishes rather than a particular food. The foods that fall into any one of these categories can vary all the way from low fat, low calorie, and high fiber, to the complete opposite! If you base your assessment of your eating habits on such food generalizations, you could wind up way off in your estimates of your calorie or fat intake. And this is just the type of mistake that could explain why you don't lose weight, or lower your cholesterol, when you think you should!

Food Inattentiveness

The third pitfall has to do with eating—without paying attention! We almost always pay attention to meals. That is, we really "register" that we are eating at mealtime because all other activity tends to stop. But food on the run, food during other recreational activity, and intermittent snacks often go overlooked, and unreported, even to ourselves!

Personally, I am always inclined to think of pistachios. I cannot recall a single patient over the past fifteen years who ever reported on a dietary intake form, or in discussing their diet, their intake of pistachios. But I happen to know that some of my patients have occasionally eaten a pistachio or two! I think pistachios are an inattentiveness food *par excellence*. They are small, eaten just a few at a time, and often while doing other things. So they go unnoticed while the calories, perhaps quite a few, are duly recorded at our waistlines. This sort of oversight pertains to many snack foods, and drinks, not just pistachios. The more this happens, the less the eating habits we report will reflect reality, and the less our estimates will provide meaningful guidance to our weight-control efforts.

Some Easily Overlooked Sources of Calories

SOURCE	CALORIES
Coffee creamer (Half & Half) and sugar for one cup of coffee	66
Butter for one bagel (2 pats)	72
Cream cheese for one bagel (3 Tbsp.)	153
One beer	146
One glass of wine	84
One "handful" (one-half cup) of pistachios	365
12 oz. regular soda	152

Overestimating Energy Expenditure

Another challenge to accurate assessments of the balance between calories consumed, and calories used, is the common tendency to overestimate how many calories were used. Energy is expended in three ways: resting (basal) metabolism, physical activity, and the generation of heat after eating (called *postprandial thermogenesis* or the "thermic effect of food"). In general, basal metabolism accounts for about 70 percent of energy expenditure, and physical activity and thermogenesis for about 15 percent each.

Calories burned in a variety of activities are shown on page 296.

Doing the Metabolism Math (Am I Thin Yet?)

By considering how our calories are generally used, you will probably realize that you tend to overestimate the calories you use up in physical activity. Here is an example.

It's Not My Food!

Amy, thirty-four, has three kids, ages three, six, and eight. The three-and six-year-old are fussy eaters. They tend to leave a lot of food on their plates. Having grown up with, "There are people starving in China!" Amy can't stand to "waste" food—so she eats it instead. But she tends to overlook the miscellaneous leftovers of her kids' food when she considers her own eating habits. After all, that's not really her food. The trouble is, it adds up to several hundred calories to her typical day.

Consider that you walk briskly for a full hour every day of the week. This is a considerable commitment to exercise, and one not all of us can match. Walking briskly increases energy expenditure 4 to 5 times over the basal rate. Assume that the basal rate is 1.5 kcal/min (the actual basal rate varies with many factors, such as body size, so any value used is a rough estimate). At rest, this basal rate would result in the use of 90 kcal in an hour, 1.5 kcal per minute, multiplied by 60 minutes.

By walking briskly, and increasing from 1.5 to 6 kcal/min, a total of 360 kcal would be burned in the same hour, 6 kcal per minute, multiplied by 60 minutes. The difference between calories burned at rest during that hour (90) and calories burned by walking briskly during that same hour (360) is 270 calories (360 minus 90).

This represents the calories burned due to walking, and in terms of a weight-loss attempt, would represent the net "benefit" of walking one hour per day. You may think that this level of energy expenditure should lead to weight loss, but it probably would not. Here's why.

A Pound of Flesh

A pound equals 454 grams. A pound of body fat, therefore, has 454 grams of fat. Each gram of fat has 9 kcal. Thus, a pound of fat has approximately 4,000 kcal (454 multiplied by 9). In order to lose, or burn, a pound of fat, we need to use up roughly 4,000 kcal more than we take in.

If you want to lose that pound of body fat over the course of a week, you need to take in thirty-five hundred to four thousand fewer calories than you burn over that same week. If you want to spread the "calorie deficit" out evenly, you need to take in five to six hundred fewer calories than you burn each day to reach you goal by week's end. If you do this, you will lose 1 lb per week.

See the problem? If you maintain your usual eating habits that keep your weight stable, and then start walking briskly for an hour every day, you are only burning enough calories to lose approximately 1/2 lb per week. This is not bad! But it will probably be disappointing when it happens to you. You expect more benefit from so much effort. You may get frustrated, and give up. Then, it's back to the weight-loss drawing board.

Misconstruing Fat for Calories

Another common pitfall is the tendency to think that low-fat foods are low-calorie foods. In general, reducing fat intake does lead to reduced calorie intake. But low-calorie foods high in sugar or processed carbohydrates can be eaten in excess, and make up for the calories removed with the fat. In fact, many people feel free to eat as much as they want when they see "low fat" on a food label, and may do more than compensate for the calories removed, actually eating more!

Nutrition Surprise

If you are working to improve your diet or control your weight, you will likely pay fairly close attention to the foods you choose. But then there are the surprises, totally unexpected additions to your daily diet due to well-intentioned coworkers ("I brought bagels!"), parties ("You simply *must* have a slice of cake; it's his birthday!"), holidays, meetings, and so on. With food as the focal point of most of our social interactions, the "unexpected" addition to your diet can be expected to come along quite frequently, and in the process may cause your total intake of calories, and your dietary pattern overall, to be quite different than you intended.

The Eat Out Fake-out

Yet another difficulty in assessing actual dietary intake arises if you often eat outside your home. Restaurants can be quite misleading in what they reveal on a menu. Unless you interrogate your server or eat at a restaurant you know very well, you might order pasta and vegetables, never aware of the cream sauce; or broiled fish, uninformed of the butter bathing it.

Eating Under the Influence (of Something Other than Hunger!)

Then, there is that misperception that we eat because we're hungry! Of course, we sometimes do, although with food so readily available so much of the time, many people in the modern world almost never know true hunger. But food is eaten for many reasons other than even the subtle, early pangs of hunger, such as stress, boredom, anxiety, frustration, celebration, solidarity, and so on. Many of these acts of "unhungry ingestion" go overlooked.

Disparity Disbelief

Most of us, even though we've known since we were kids that life isn't always fair, really wish it were! So, when we process information about the world, we tend to do it in a way that imposes a certain sense of fairness. If you, for example, know one or more people who can eat whatever they want and not gain weight, you likely perceive that as "unfair," if you struggle to control your own weight. The unfairness of it takes on a life of its own, and your ability to assess disparities between your diet and theirs, your activity level and theirs, may be impaired. You may believe they eat more than you, but it might not be true. Thus, there may be actual disparities that you simply stop seeing or believing are there in order to reconcile reality with your perception of it.

Little White Lies

Because we all want to eat well, be lean, be healthy, it's nice to hear, and tempting to believe, that we are doing a great job—whether or not we actually are. Because we live in a society where so few people eat well, where few adults are physically active, and where a majority is overweight, "doing a great job" is relative. So if we take any modest measures to improve dietary patterns or weight, we are likely to have them exaggerated back at us by family and friends.

The exaggeration comes in one of two forms, usually: genuine praise and undercover sabotage. The genuine praise comes from those who are impressed with your efforts (even if you, in fact, are not), and represents a blend of support and a positive kind of envy. Remember, more than half of U.S. adults are overweight, so most people on the sidelines of your weight-control effort have cause to be thinking about their own.

The undercover sabotage is so subtle that the "perpetrator" may well be unaware of it. It will come in the form of, "*You* don't need to lose any *more* weight!" or, "Just *one* slice couldn't hurt!" or, "If you keep this up, you'll be *too* thin!" just to name a few variations on the theme. Well intentioned or otherwise, these generally inaccurate, sideline assessments of your dietary discipline are often the product of the commentator's own struggles, and their difficulty in seeing you succeed. Note that this tendency to sabotage is very common, and does not imply a bad streak; you may have practiced it yourself on someone else!

If You Are What You Eat, Then What the Heck Are You?

Now, in light of these considerations, and perhaps many others that come readily to your mind, you will need to acknowledge that gaining an accurate appraisal of your diet may not be so simple. In fact, it's quite challenging—even for professionals. At the population level, nutrition researchers continue to struggle with means of reliably gauging dietary intake in the U.S. Food frequency questionnaires tend to over-report intake; dietary recalls tend to under-report; food diaries are very labor intensive and still subject to inaccuracies; metabolic ward studies are very expensive and inconvenient. Fortunately for you, you can leave the challenge of tracking national dietary patterns to the researchers and nutrition professionals. Your mission at the moment is to gain an accurate assessment of just one diet: yours.

To know where you are, so you can better gauge where you need to go, you must be willing to take an honest and thorough dietary inventory. There are tools to help you do the job well. The simplest is a food diary, in which you record, for several days, a week, or more, everything you're eating, along with when, where, and even why.

That's Some Coffee!

I recently saw a patient who wanted to lose weight very badly, and simply hadn't been able to do so. She brought in a food diary that showed that she was drinking as many as six cups of coffee each day, each with two packets of sugar and a tablespoon of cream. That's a total of forty-six calories from the sugar and another thirty from the cream in each cup—for six cups, that's 456 calories per day! Simply by substituting a low-calorie sweetener and nonfat powdered milk, almost all of those calories could be eliminated. That would be enough to lose a pound a week, and we hadn't even gotten past the coffee to the food! Your food diary may provide you with similar revelations.

Taking Inventory

We recommend that you reproduce the food diary chart on page 236 and use it to record everything that you eat and drink for as many days as you are willing over the next two weeks. Be sure to include days that represent your usual eating habits, and to include both work and non-work days, weekdays, and weekends. Note what you ate; an estimate of the portion size; when you ate (time); where you ate or the source of the food (e.g., home, car, restaurant, office, vending machine, etc.); and why, whether for hunger, boredom, stress relief, or some other reason.

Know Thy Diet

Just filling out the diary will doubtless bring things to your attention that you had previously not considered. But there is much more that you can do. You may want to analyze your dietary intake so that you truly know the calories, fat, sugar, fiber, or salt in your typical day or week. This can be done with the help of a dietitian, or on your own using the Internet (check out: www.dietwatch.com, www.webdietitian .com, or www.eDiets.com), or nutrition analysis software. Guidance for approaching this either way, or both, is offered in Section IV. Even without a full nutritional analysis, you can of course review your food diary with a dietitian, doctor, or other professional to identify both what you should change to improve your diet, and how you can implement recommended changes successfully.

From Here, Getting There

Compare the food diary and analysis to the diet recommended throughout this book to see where you come closest to a healthful pattern, and where you deviate from it the most. This can help define the areas where your effort at dietary modification should be concentrated. You will also gain insight into the particular foods, food groups, and nutrient classes that are most likely causing you any trouble you are having with weight control or other diet-related health issues.

All about Eating

The diary, and its analysis, can provide you with a great deal more useful information. Turn your attention now to the where/when/why responses. Are there particular places where you tend to struggle most with your diet? Are you subject to certain "environmental cues" that cause you to eat less well than you would like? Are there times of day that seem to be your "vulnerable" times? Are there clear reasons other than hunger why you eat? Are there particular foods you tend to eat in response to particular emotions or situations?

You can probably tell just by considering this list of questions how powerful, and empowering, the answers are likely to be. There may be many influences on your dietary pattern that you have taken for granted or never considered. This exercise will cause you to find them, define them, and consider their importance.

You have rounded out the knowledge required to eat well if you have reconsidered yourself in the context of evolutionary biology, reaffirmed what you probably already knew, but now know with complete conviction about healthful eating, and made diligent and candid assessments of your starting diet: its *whats*, its *whens*, its *wheres*, and its *whys*. With this knowledge in place, you have taken step one along the *way to eat*, and should be ready to acquire the empowering skills of behavior modification provided in Section II.

Section Two:

Power

Knowledge is like a lever used to lift a heavy object; the force to do the lifting must still be applied. The more reasons you have for eating as you now do, the more reasons you will need to change how you eat, and the heavier the lifting required!

The force, or power, to improve the way you eat forever is the science of behavior change. Knowledge tells you "what," power is "how." Ready for some power? Right this way...

Step 2:

Meet the Challenge of Change

CHANGING ALMOST ANY behavior is difficult. The reason for this has to do with why change is needed or wanted. The way we behave is a choice we make based on many competing influences. In some sense, we weigh the pros and cons of all of the available choices and settle on a particular pattern of behavior. To change to a new pattern of behavior, any new pattern, requires that we, at least partially, abandon the pattern we chose in the first place. This is difficult because any change requires giving up the familiar, which is generally preferred to the unfamiliar. And it is simply difficult because starting something new is rarely the path of least resistance. Just as getting a heavy object to start moving across the floor is more difficult than keeping it moving, initiating change is tough.

Our behavioral, or lifestyle, choices include a great many things other than diet, but diet is among the most important behavioral choices each of us makes. Despite the fact that we do choose our lifestyle, we may not behave in a manner that makes us entirely happy. But even if you are not entirely happy with your diet—in fact, even if you are rather unhappy with it—you need to acknowledge that you chose it. You could be eating some other way: more, less, or just different. But you are not—you are eating precisely what and how you are eating!

While there are a great many influences on your dietary pattern that you do not control, the pattern itself represents an interaction between you and those influences. So, your priorities are an important part of the equation. Therefore, the dietary pattern you have chosen reflects something about the way you want to be eating.

Therein lies the challenge of behavior change. All of the factors that led to the choice of a particular behavior or behavioral pattern in the first place lie in your way when you try to change. This doesn't mean change is impossibly difficult, but it does mean that it's not as simple as one might hope. You cannot simply want to change, or decide to change, and effortlessly assume some new dietary pattern. You must anticipate the challenges you will face.

When the Going Gets Tough, the Smart Get Science

Experts in behavior modification generally acknowledge that diet is particularly difficult to change. While smoking cessation is hard to do, the decision itself is simple: yes, or no. The same is true for many behaviors, from alcohol and drug use to physical activity. Diet does not allow for a "just say yes" or "no" approach, however. Food is essential for survival, and cannot be avoided, yet imposes considerable risks as well. To navigate successfully between the risks and benefits of diet requires particularly clever use of the very best theories that behavior modification science has to offer. Elements of several of the most widely used and respected behavior change models are combined to help you set out on the *way to eat*.

Health and Behavior from the Health Institute in Washington, D.C., defines these behavior change models, which we adapted for *The Way to Eat*:

- The *Transtheoretical Model* includes the stages of change, processes of change, and elements of other theories, and asserts that behavior change progresses through predictable stages, and that needs vary by stage.
- *Social Cognitive Theory* emphasizes the role of expected outcomes, locus of control, and efficacy, or ability. Self-efficacy refers to one's belief in their ability to initiate change; locus of control refers to one's belief that outcomes will be affected by behavior.
- The *Health Beliefs Model* asserts in essence that behavior change relates to one's personal perception of risk, benefit, and opportunity.

Getting Down to Basics

Some very simple considerations can help put the power of behavior change theory and science in your hands.

Consider that you have received or sought advice about dietary change before. In fact, you probably know what you should do. You have heard the rumors that fruits, vegetables, and grains are good for your health, and you should be physically active. And since you want the benefits to appearance and health that these changes would provide, you are motivated to modify your diet and activity level. Yet you do not. Or if you do, the changes you make are short-lived, much like New Year's resolutions. Then you return to your previous diet and activity pattern. Why?

Because motivation is only half of what determines behavior and the efforts to change it. The other half is the difficulty involved, the resistance to change we do not control.

Where There's a Will...There's a Will

Will alone is not enough; there's got to be a reasonable way! Each impediment to healthy eating in the modern world contributes something to the cumulative difficulty you face in efforts to change your diet, to control your weight, to improve your health. When the sum of all this difficulty exceeds your motivation, no matter how great your motivation, you will not, cannot, change your behavior. Worse still, failing to change your behavior despite a strong motivation to do so leaves you feeling terribly frustrated, even discouraged. If you don't eat as you should, if you are overweight, both you and others are apt to think that it is your fault. But if you are already motivated to change, blaming yourself, or being blamed by others, for an inability to do so is worse than not helpful; it is outright harmful. The proverbial case of kicking someone who is down, such victim blaming generates feelings of failure, eroding the motivation and self-efficacy necessary for any future, and ultimately successful, attempts at behavior change.

All too often ignored in efforts to improve health through behavior change are the barriers to that change. A schedule that does not readily accommodate exercise may outweigh your motivation to be physically active. The convenience and familiarity of fast food, and uncertainty about how to change patterns of shopping and cooking, may triumph over your desire to improve your diet. Even if motivation is fairly high, change cannot occur if resistance to change is higher.

I think often of a patient I have known for years, whom we will call Linda. Linda is a wonderful woman. Now in her early 70s, she is a loving wife, mother, and grandmother. She is intelligent, active, vivacious, and interesting.

But for all the time I've known her, Linda has tended to sum herself up in just one word: fat. The work we have done together has resulted in a weight loss of eighteen pounds, maintenance of that loss for years now, and Linda beats up on herself less than she did before. But, I am sorry to say, after literally decades of blaming herself for her inability to control her weight and be as thin as she would like, the scars left behind are very tenacious. Linda certainly knows I don't think her weight problem is her fault. And she has come to know that herself. But feeling it is quite another matter.

Overcoming the various obstacles to dietary change would be enough of a challenge if that were all that were required. But if you are discouraged by prior, unsuccessful attempts to change your diet, the biggest obstacle of all is likely to be…you! If you feel defeated, if your self-esteem has taken a beating, you don't have the self-efficacy you need to undertake change. You may still want to change, but there is no force to carry you along. You are "blown away" by the unrelenting resistance you have tried to confront.

What Weighs You Down

Assuming you want to lose weight, you should realize that the loss of several pounds is actually far less important than giving up the weighty burden of feeling as if you've failed. If your prior efforts to improve your diet or control your weight have been unsuccessful, you are not to blame. But as long as you think you are, you are weighed down. If you have been unable to change your diet before, you must forgive yourself; it was no more your fault than your inability to fly like a bird or breathe under water like a fish. Forgive yourself, and you can set down the heavy burden of disappointment, self-recrimination, or shame—far heavier than any amount of body fat. Set these down, and the winds of change will start to carry you.

The Winds of Change

Just as wind always blows from high pressure to low pressure, behavior, too, is controlled by two simple and opposing forces: the desire to change, or motivation, and the resistance to change, or difficulty. When resistance equals or exceeds motivation, change is prevented; when motivation exceeds resistance, change occurs. Increases or decreases in the force of either motivation or resistance can either be the basis for change or a barrier to it.

Maximize Your Motivation

The word "motivation" has the same Latin root as "motion"; both refer to the capacity to change place, or get going. In the case of behavior, the pertinent change is from one pattern to another. Motivation is the force that initiates such a change. Superficially, motivation is a lot like desire. If you want to change your diet, you are motivated to do so. But because motivation refers to the force underlying actual movement, it is more complex and subtle than simply wanting.

Accounting for Change

Most behaviors that make up our lifestyle are selected without a great deal of conscious consideration. It is very doubtful that you have compiled charts and graphs to characterize the relative pros and cons of sleeping less or more, working harder or less hard, exercising or not, eating one way or another. But you have, in fact, processed these very same pros and cons without being conscious of it.

You probably know that sleeping eight hours a night is good for your health. But if you sleep less than that, it is because you are willing to give up the health benefits of more sleep for some alternative benefits (or because you have insomnia). Perhaps by sleeping only six hours a night you can be more productive professionally, or spend more time with your children, or find the time to keep your house in order. At some level, you have weighed the advantages and disadvantages of one choice against another, and settled on the one that maximizes your "benefit" relative to "cost." Another way of describing cost and benefit is "utility," or usefulness. We tend to choose behaviors that give us the most utility.

The implication of lifestyle choice being the product of this almost accidental "utility analysis" is that motivation can be going in several directions at once. You can be motivated to quit smoking, and motivated to smoke. You can be motivated to change your diet, and motivated to maintain it. And you probably are!

Motivation is Relative

Consider that your current dietary pattern was a choice you made. As discussed in Section III, this choice has been influenced by a great many factors not under your control. Nonetheless, what you eat, compared to anyone else, and compared to the other options available to you, is what you choose to eat. There must be reasons for the choice, even if you have not given them a great deal of thought. While eating less might lead to weight loss, eating more may be more satisfying. While eating more fruits and vegetables might promote health, eating chocolate feels really good! And so on. Motivation was part of the process that led to your current dietary pattern. For this reason, simply wanting to change cannot be enough to effect change. For movement to occur, the force of wanting to change must exceed the force of wanting to remain where you are.

Making Up (With) Your Mind

As the saying goes, honesty is the best policy. This is certainly true in behavior change. If you attempt to change a behavior, particularly one as challenging as your eating habits, without a ruthlessly honest appraisal of your motivation, you may wind up disappointed. The process of measuring motivation that tends to work well is the construction of a *decision balance*.

A decision balance is simply a table in which you list all of the anticipated advantages of making a change, along with the disadvantages of doing so. It can be kept this simple, just two choices or "cells," or expanded to include the advantages of not making a change, along with the disadvantages of that choice. A decision balance for dietary change can relate to a complete overhaul of your diet, or to a particular step in improving your diet, such as reducing your fat or sodium intake.

Should I Stay or Should I Go?
A Decision Balance for Changing Dietary Pattern
with Hypothetical Entries

Changing	Staying the Same
Advantages	**Advantages**
Weight loss	Easy
Better health	Can eat favorite foods
More energy	
Disadvantages	**Disadvantages**
Hard work	No weight loss
Giving up sweets	No health benefits
Hunger	Possible weight gain

Your Decisions, in the Balance

A decision balance may be created for any behavior change you are considering. The balance is most useful when the change represents a toss-up, when the motivation level for change and the motivation level for maintenance of the status quo are very close. Simply by constructing the balance and reviewing it, you may find the additional motivation needed to make the change of interest. Alternatively, of course, your balance may lead to just the opposite conclusion: that the cold, hard facts favor maintaining your current diet!

When you want to change, but your decision balance does not seem to favor change, there are two implications. The first is that your balance is incomplete, that you have left out some of the advantages of change, or disadvantages of not changing. The other implication is that your balance is correct, but needs to be altered before it will support a decision to change.

One of the ways of altering the content of a decision balance is to acquire new skills that make change easier, or learn new information that makes the appeal of change greater. If you can find new items to add to the *advantages of change* or the *disadvantages of not changing,* or if you can remove some of the *disadvantages of changing* or *advantages of not changing*, your balance will lead to a new conclusion. The real value of the decision balance is that it shows you the truth about your motivation, and guides you both to what you need and to a realistic assessment of your readiness for change.

Counting Reasons for Change

If you find the decision balance useful, you may want to take it one step further and devise a *quantitative decision balance*. The simple list of pros and cons of change versus maintenance may not allow you to assess your motivation adequately, because some of the items may matter more to you than others.

To account for this, you could assign a "weight" to the items in your balance, such as a score from 1 to 5. Low priority items could receive a 1, and highest priority items a 5. To determine if your entries favor change or not, add the scores for the advantages of change to the scores for the disadvantages of not changing (A). Then add the scores for the disadvantages of change to the scores for the advantages of not changing (B). If A is more than B, the balance favors a change now. If B equals, or is more than A, more motivation for change is required to make a dietary change that is likely to succeed.

Even a quantitative decision balance does not guarantee a completely accurate assessment of your effective motivation. You might have forgotten some item, such as the benefits to your self-esteem of changing your diet, or the extra time you will need to spend shopping until you get used to your new way of eating. Whenever you come upon some new consideration that affects your motivation, you can add it to your balance so that it remains current as your insight increases.

Each time you enter a new item into a decision balance, you have a clearer and more complete picture of your motivation. The balance that ultimately serves as your basis for change may take shape right away, or may require multiple revisions. Either is fine—both represent part of the process of change. You are on your way, and that's what matters.

Your Personal Pep Rally

A few simple strategies can help you maximize your motivation:

- *Acknowledging Ambivalence:* Use a decision balance to make an honest appraisal of why you might want not to change, even though you also want to change.
- *Confronting Discrepancies:* Assess the ways in which the outcomes you want, and your behavior, may be at odds.
- *Rolling with Resistance:* Learn from obstacles encountered as you try to change your diet; don't let them discourage you.
- *Supporting Self-efficacy:* Keep in mind that the more strategies you learn, the more capable you become of lasting change; be patient, and stay confident.
- *Positive Imaging:* Picture the desirable outcomes successfully changing your behavior will help you achieve.
- *Negative Imaging:* Picture the undesirable outcomes successfully changing your behavior will help you leave behind.
- *Modeling:* Follow a good example set by someone else.
- *Reinforcement:* Reward yourself for sticking to your commitments.
- *Social Contracting:* Tell a confidante about your plans, and ask them to help keep you on track.
- *Social Support:* Get others to join you in your behavior change effort, and support one another.

Buoyed along by both your own motivation and that of friends and family working to support you, you begin to have the necessary power to turn your knowledge of healthful eating into your way of eating for life. By gaining insight into the importance of barriers to change, and of converting these obstacles into opportunity, your power to change becomes much greater still.

Reduce Resistance

In the immortal words of the Rolling Stones, "You can't always get what you want." There is, funny enough, a certain wisdom in that simple statement that gets at some of the subtle challenges of behavior modification. Wanting to change behavior is not, and cannot be, enough—

Retail Reinforcement

One of the things Janet, age fifty-two, likes even better than a hot cinnamon bun or luscious slice of cake is a nice wardrobe. To help keep herself motivated to eat well, Janet puts aside a small amount of money—ten or twenty dollars—whenever she successfully resists a strong temptation to give up her good eating habits. She then uses the savings to buy some nice clothes from time to time, which provides further motivation to her to make sure she continues to fit into them! You, too, should use rewards that work well for you to maximize and maintain your motivation.

---

or everyone wanting to change their behavior would do so. A lot more people have wanted to climb Mt. Everest than have done so.

Some have done so, however, but not just because they wanted to. They also did a pretty good job of sizing up the obstacle they faced: a great, big, cold, harsh mountain of rock and ice and snow. A thorough understanding of the obstacle, and of the skills, techniques, and strategies needed to surmount it, coupled with their desire and will, got them to the summit. Their power to succeed comes both from motivation and the means to overcome resistance—from having not just the *will*, but also a *way*.

Barriers, Within & Without

The barriers to eating well relate to many factors and influences. Our Stone Age physiologies are well designed to keep us going in a world of constant physical activity and limited food. But the very features that promote survival in such a world create great vulnerability in the modern world. And, because these vulnerabilities are built into our metabolism and physiology, they are completely involuntary, not under our control. These are barriers to our efforts at eating well. We can either know them, prepare for them, and overcome them, or come upon them by surprise and have them block our path. But they cannot be avoided; they are part of us. To use a time-honored witticism, we have met the enemy, and it is us!

Social influences, cultural influences, environmental conditions, and industry practices compound the vulnerabilities of metabolism. The food industry exists to sell us food, so it tailors its products and its messages to maximize the temptation into which we are drawn. Advertising exploits our beliefs, our hopes, and our cravings. A culture that has always valued food provides little guidance to our efforts at restraint. A complex, intricate network of influences, internal and external, stands between us and our dietary health goals.

Of Obstacles & Opportunities

Are you thinking this is bad news? Feeling discouraged? Don't!

Actually, this is excellent news. The barriers to eating well are there, whether you know about them or not. If you do not know about them, if you are not forewarned, then you cannot be forearmed. You will encounter resistance whether you expect it or not; you will encounter your foe whether or not you anticipate doing so, and know who your foe is. If you have made prior attempts to improve your diet or control your weight without success or satisfaction, these unanticipated barriers are very likely the reason why.

But with foreknowledge of resistance, of what and where the barriers are, you can navigate around them, over them, and past them. And even better. In what you may want to consider *behavior change alchemy*, just by knowing what obstacles you face, you can convert obstacles into opportunities. Each obstacle to eating well is an invitation to learn something about dietary health, human physiology, or environmental influences.

The Way Less Traveled

Seeing obstacles as opportunities sets you up to succeed in ways never before possible. As you layer strategy upon strategy, skill upon skill, you become stronger, more resilient, and more resourceful. You become, essentially, an expert in navigating the hazards of the modern nutritional world. And as an expert, you come to find that the "resistance" of the nutritional environment cannot resist you!

This view, this approach, goes well beyond the fifty-four common barriers to eating well addressed in the next four Steps. It applies just as well to the obstacles you encounter that are unique to you, or even to a particular situation. The strategies you learn are like the vocabulary of a new language. Once you speak it fluently, you are no longer limited to the sentences you have been taught; you can combine words in limitless combinations, in your own particular way.

The Way, Behind & Ahead

You have taken two key steps forward. Having done so, bring your knowledge and power, your will and capacity to change, to Section III, where you will acquire the many skills and strategies that will make you unstoppable on your way to a lifetime of dietary health, weight control, and contentment with food.

Section Three:

The Way!

More than half of all adults in the United States, and rising percentages in all industrialized countries, are overweight or obese. Countless millions are preoccupied with food, frustrated with their inability to eat the way they feel they should, and unhappy with their health or appearance. The modern world is experiencing a nutrition crisis.

A Dangerous Opportunity

There is just one word, or character, in Chinese for both danger and opportunity: the word that translates to *crisis*. There is considerable wisdom in viewing a crisis in general, and our nutritional crisis specifically, as a dangerous opportunity.

Every aspect of the nutritional environment that contributes to poor eating habits is a danger that, if understood and addressed, can be used to help us eat well. The obstacles to healthful eating may be viewed as something else altogether: opportunities.

Fundamentally, we are all threatened by the challenges of the modern environment. The constant temptations of excessive sugar, salt, and fat are compounded by the conveniences of modern society and the resultant, progressive decline in our physical activity levels. In short, we live in a nutritional environment that is largely at odds with our needs for healthful eating. Adding to the challenges of our metabolism and taste preferences are folklore, cultural norms, social pressures, media messages, industry practices, and the complicated psychology of eating for reasons other than hunger.

This array of obstacles to healthful eating is intimidating at first. But when the barriers to eating well are understood, they become less danger and more opportunity. Ignoring these barriers makes dietary change very nearly impossible—like trying to get through an obstacle course with your eyes closed! Time to open your eyes.

On the Brink of Change

This section reveals the many potential barriers to eating well and demonstrates how each is, in fact, an opportunity. But it serves another purpose as well. If you have previously attempted dietary change, or weight loss, and have not succeeded—and if what you've read so far has not convinced you to forgive yourself yet—this section may do the job. Each time you read about an "obstacle" you didn't know was there, or didn't know was important, or didn't know how to surmount, ask yourself, *"How could I have succeeded without knowing this*? How could I hope to cross an obstacle course with my eyes closed?" As that question is repeated, you should feel the weight of past "failures" fall from you.

The knowledge of where you are and where you're going, the power of initiating change and setting your new diet in motion, and the buoyancy of forgiveness should all come together. Add to these a "map" that shows the route, the skills, and the strategies to overcome obstacles, and the attitude that accepts each obstacle as an opportunity, and what's to stop you?! Nothing!

Alike, but Different

Each of us is unique, but we are also much alike. While some of the challenges you face on your way to eating well are doubtless unique to you, most are shared with the rest of us. Included in these four Steps are fifty-four potential obstacles to healthful eating and the strategies for dealing with each. You will see some strategies repeated, because they can be used to deal with more than one barrier. You don't need to learn a completely unique set of strategies or skills to overcome each obstacle.

Just as Step 1 pointed out that the same basic dietary pattern can lead you toward the many health and weight goals you might have, so, too, a small range of basic strategies can lead you toward that dietary pattern.

Step 3:

Conquer Your Cravings & Master Your Metabolism!

THE COMPOSITION OF our prehistoric food supply is important to the type of food we are adapted to eat. Our metabolism and our physiology—the very ways in which our bodies function—developed partly in response to the things our ancestors ate. Knowing this provides powerful insights into our preferences, our traits and tendencies, our cravings and aversions, our strengths, and our vulnerabilities.

These insights are the basis for a powerful array of skills and strategies that convert the potential obstacles of a prehistoric metabolism into opportunities for nutritional health. This step characterizes the strategies needed to surmount the many potential barriers to healthful eating that are built into our metabolism, barriers that reside within our very genetic makeup, which you likely did not even know were there. Yet these are among the forces which influence your eating most profoundly because, quite simply, these barriers are a part of you, a part of us all—built into our metabolism.

The obstacles you will encounter and learn to overcome in this step include:

1) Addictive Properties of Dietary Fat
2) Discomfort/Inconvenience Associated with
    Changes to a High-fiber Diet
3) Fear of Hunger
4) Innate Preference for Sugar

> 5) *Persistent Appetite (Leptin Resistance)*
> 6) *Thrifty Metabolism (Insulin Resistance)*
> 7) *Normal/Natural Tendency to Binge Eat*
> 8) *Normal Preference for Familiar Foods;*
>   *Distaste for Unfamiliar Foods*
> 9) *Normal/Natural Preference for Salt*
> 10) *Pleasure/Gratification Induced by Food*
> 11) *Sensory Specific Satiety*
> 12) *Variations in Basal Metabolism*
> 13) *Variations in Body Type/Fat Deposition*
> 14) *Variations in Taste Sensitivity*
> 15) *Weight Loss Plateau*

Obstacle/Opportunity 1
Addictive Properties of Dietary Fat

There is scientific evidence that eating sugar and fat may stimulate pleasure at the same body receptors (opioid receptors) that respond to the drug morphine, and to our own endorphins, the chemicals responsible for the famous "runner's high." Eating fat stimulates the opioid receptors, making dietary fat if not actually addictive, then at least alarmingly close. This is not a matter of choice; it's built right into our cells.

The Then/Now Conflict

Our prehistoric preference for fat makes sense. For our ancestors, dietary fat was scarce, yet a vital source of essential nutrients and energy. Almost all natural food sources—plant and animal—available to our ancestors were low in fat. The exceptions were organ meats, bone marrow, and cholesterol-rich foods such as eggs. Our ancestors needed fat in their diet because fatty acids are required components of our cell membranes. Essential fatty acids are required nutrients for human health. And, of course, the energy density of fat would make it very valuable to people always working hard to get enough food energy to survive. Given all of these circumstances, it follows almost intuitively that our ancestors would have acquired a taste for fat that became a built-in aspect of our metabolism over the eons.

The modern world, however, provides an overabundance of fat-rich fast food, meats, dairy products, and processed foods of many varieties. When combined with this plentiful supply, our Stone Age "fat addiction" creates an important challenge to eating well and controlling calorie intake.

Strategy

As with many, indeed most, of the barriers to eating well, the successful approach to this one begins with knowing it exists. You are likely aware that certain foods are hard to resist. Your "weakness" may be cake or ice cream, cheese or bacon, chips and dips, cold cuts, steak, or fried chicken. Perhaps it's all of these. However you would compose your list, it would likely contain many foods rich in fat. Knowing that these fat-rich foods are calorie-rich foods, and potentially hazardous to your health if consumed excessively, you may have tried to avoid them, or at least limit your intake. And when these efforts failed, or when you gave them up entirely, you may have felt as if you failed, as if you did not have sufficient willpower or resolve. And you have doubtless complained that if it tastes good, it's never good for you, and if it's good for you, it invariably tastes less good!

Now you know that willpower was never the issue. Rather, you have been programmed to like fat in your diet. In fact, you have been designed to get "addicted" to it! Addiction is a physical dependence on something that interacts with our bodies in a way that reinforces the need for it.

Fat Makes Fat

Unfortunately, the modern nutritional environment provides the very varieties of fat (saturated and trans) most harmful to health. Because we are all exposed to so much fatty food, most of us eat it all the time. This increases our familiarity with, and preference for, high-fat foods, because familiarity is another factor influencing our dietary preferences. Thus, the more fat we eat, the more we want. Because it is so energy dense, fat in the diet contributes disproportionately to calorie intake; high-fat diets are typically high-energy diets, and thus tend to lead to weight gain.

Know and Select Foods Naturally Low in Fat

One key component of a winning strategy for reducing fat intake is to know the foods that are naturally low in fat, and to shift from high-fat to low-fat foods. Fruits, vegetables, and grains are low in fat, and for a variety of reasons, a diet based primarily on these foods promotes health. Eating such foods regularly reduces fat and calories, with no need to analyze fat content. Whenever you are eating fruits, vegetables, or whole grains that have not been processed, you are eating low-fat foods.

Getting Pleasure from What You Don't Eat

Naturally, the apple or whole-grain bagel or nonfat yogurt you eat instead of a cinnamon bun dripping with butter may be, especially at first, less intensely pleasurable. While that may seem like a sacrifice, consider it in context. You may be dissatisfied with your weight, cholesterol, blood pressure, or blood sugar. Whatever your concern, it is a source of discontent, or anxiety, or sorrow. So the pleasure you get from your current diet is offset by the displeasure you get from some of its consequences.

By substituting that apple for that cinnamon bun, you trade a certain amount of immediate gratification for a certain amount of delayed gratification. If the delayed gratification is greater, this is not a sacrifice, but rather an investment. The investment is most challenging at the start. Very soon, the new pattern becomes a part of your routine. You don't think about the cinnamon bun, and thus don't miss it. Besides which, once you really do establish a good eating pattern that is relatively low in fat, an occasional cinnamon bun is fine, if it still appeals.

Fun Instead of Fat!

Another important Strategy is to find time and occasion to enjoy yourself. Part of what makes dietary fat so irresistible is the fact that it gives pleasure. A good defense against its lure is to replace the pleasure it provides. Some of this pleasure can come from food. Some can come from anything else you like and can find time to do, the best examples being physically active pursuits that provide the added benefit of exercise. If possible, for example, take a portable, low-fat lunch and go for a walk outside on a beautiful day, rather than eating a high-fat lunch at your desk. Listen to music you like, take a warm bath, play some basketball: whatever! Combine the pleasure you get from food with some pleasure you get from alternatives to food.

Get by with a Little Help from Your Friends

A simple strategy of great potential help as you tackle many of the challenges to eating well is to ask for help from friends, family, and coworkers. Be quite explicit. Let everyone in your social support network know you are trying to reduce your intake of fat because "_____" (you fill in the blank), that it's hard, and that you would very much appreciate help and support.

John Donne said, "No man is an island," and in efforts at dietary health, none of us can create a nutritional oasis all on our own, either. Ask for the help you need. And consider going even one step further: encourage your friends or family or coworkers to join you as you work to cut back on your fat intake, and share the strategies that you find most helpful.

Get the Food Facts

To go further in efforts at controlling fat intake requires that you attend to food labels. Detailed guidance in food label interpretation is provided in Section IV.

Overall, a fat intake of not more than 30 percent of total calories is recommended. We consider a fat intake of between 20 and 25 percent of calories even better. Eating lots of natural foods—fruit, vegetables, and grains—will help you get closer to this goal. The next step is to reduce the fat content of the other foods you eat.

You may want to keep track of your fat and calorie intake for a while as you get used to a low-fat way of eating. But let's be honest: counting calories and fat is pretty tedious. To minimize the need for this, you can simply familiarize yourself with the low-fat alternatives in different categories of food. Once you know which pasta sauces, breads, crackers, snacks, soups, and so on, are low in fat, you can select them on sight. Section IV provides all the help you'll need to make this transition, with guidance for shopping, reading labels, stocking your pantry, and choosing brands.

Of Fat Munching, & Number Crunching...

We recommend that less than 30 percent, preferably about 20–25 percent, of all of your calories come from fat. How can you get there without turning eating into algebra, and cooking into calculus?

Look at the calories in a serving size of any food. Then look at the grams of fat. Each gram of fat has nine calories, so multiply the grams of fat by 9. This is the number of calories from fat. Now, all you need to do is see what percentage of the calories in the serving come from fat:

[(calories from fat) / (total calories in a serving) X 100]

You don't need to add these up all day. Keep it simple: if most of the foods you eat have less than 30 percent of calories from fat, your overall diet will have less than 30 percent of calories from fat. If most of your foods are higher in fat, you don't need to do any math to know that your overall diet will also be higher in fat! So to eat well, choose wisely! No math degree required! (For more on interpreting food labels, see Section IV.)

For example, some breakfast cereals are high in fiber and low in sugar, salt, and fat. Other cereals, with often quite similar names, are high in fat, sugar, and/or salt, and low in fiber. Look for cereals that provide two or more grams of fiber per serving, and as little fat as possible, certainly not more than 25 percent of the calories. Consider this: if you eat cereal as a "healthy" component of your diet, and it provides more fat in proportion to total calories than your whole diet is supposed to provide, how likely is it that you will be able to dilute down that fat intake with other foods? Not likely. If total fat intake is to be not more than 30 percent of calories, it follows that the fat content of most foods eaten must be less than 30 percent of calories. Don't count total fat and calories, but choose the specific foods from each group wisely.

Egg pasta provides fat. Semolina pasta provides no fat, fewer calories, and more fiber. Some sauces, dressings, and spreads are high in fat; there are nonfat or low-fat alternatives to almost all of them. Don't trust the "lite" you see on the package front; it can mean many different things. Rather, look at the nutrition label and determine if the product provides 30 percent (or, better still, 20–25 percent) or less of its calories from fat. If it is higher in fat than you want your overall diet to be, look for an alternative. Some breads and crackers have added fat, others don't. Dairy products are high in fat naturally, but are available in low-fat and nonfat varieties; these are preferred. When substituting nonfat or low-fat foods for their higher-fat counterparts, remember to exercise reasonable portion control, or the calorie benefit will be lost.

The Matter of Milk

One of the most straightforward food conversions you can make to support your effort to reduce and control fat intake is from regular to skim milk. This switch is also an excellent experiment you can conduct on yourself to demonstrate that preference is driven in part by familiarity. First, you should know that whole milk provides more than 50 percent of its calories from fat; thus, it is a high-fat food. However, only 4 percent of the weight of the milk is fat, because most of the weight is water. Milk labeled 2 percent has not had 98 percent of the fat removed; it has had approximately half the fat removed. The 2 percent refers to the weight of the milk, not its calories. Nearly 30 percent of the calories in 2 percent milk are from fat; thus, it is not a low-fat food. Skim milk has had all of the fat removed.

If you are accustomed to whole milk, or even 2 percent milk, you will doubtless find skim milk watery, distasteful, and perhaps even unappetizingly bluish in color! We understand; this is quite normal. However, it is a product of your familiar diet, not a permanent stand on the part of your taste buds!

Switch to skim milk for a period of one to two weeks, and commit to that long a trial in advance. If you prefer to proceed incrementally, going from whole to 2 percent to 1 percent to skim milk, that is fine. You may also find your effort supported by use of new, "fortified" skim milk products that have added milk proteins to make them mimic the texture of fattier milk (e.g., Skim Plus, or Simply Smart).

Whatever way you choose to go, stick out the two weeks. At the end of two weeks, taste, just once, the type of milk you started with. If you

Calcium: Swimmin' in Skim...

Ounce for ounce, skim milk has much less fat than whole milk (skim milk has none), and of course many fewer calories. But it also has more calcium! The calcium in milk is dissolved in the water. The portion of milk taken up by fat has no calcium in it. The more fat, the less calcium. Fill a glass with skim, and you've also got calcium, right up to the brim!

are like most of us (I have run this experiment many times with patients, students, and friends), you will find that skim milk tastes "normal" now, and the milk you started with tastes too rich and creamy.

Once you've made this transition, it's easy to apply it to yogurt, frozen desserts, cottage cheese, etc. For coffee, try undiluted nonfat powdered milk (put the powder in first, pour the coffee over, and you don't even need to stir). It lightens the coffee the way milk does, without making it gray the way regular skim milk does! As a powder it offers the advantages of not diluting the coffee, and not cooling it down, along with long shelf-life and portability. If you drink several cups of coffee with milk each day, or eat cereal with milk in the morning, these seemingly small changes can cut significant fat and calories from your diet. An eight-ounce glass of whole milk, for example, provides 156 kcal, roughly eighty of which come from fat! In contrast, an eight-ounce glass of skim, or fat-free, milk provides 86 kcal, and no fat—while providing even more calcium.

The skim-milk conversion is a particularly clear example of how to substitute one food for another and lower your fat intake. It also shows the power of familiarity in dietary preference. These lessons can "spill" over to other foods. If you are accustomed to granola with added fat, after one to two weeks with a nonfat granola you'll like it just as much. The same is true for dressings, spreads, and sauces. Marinara sauce can provide a load of fat and calories, or almost none. Every one of these transitions you make reduces your overall fat intake, and adds one more defense against the addictive properties of dietary fat.

Make Ingredient Substitutions
There is still more you can do. After selecting foods naturally low in fat, and learning the low-fat items within the various categories of processed foods, comes ingredient substitutions. Many recipes that call for rich, high-fat sauces can be made just as readily without those ingredients. Many baked goods can be made (and remain—honest!—just as delicious) with ingredient substitutions that substantially reduce the fat and calorie content. Many such ingredients and recipe tips are provided in Section IV.

Defend the Homefront
To support your efforts at achieving and maintaining a moderate fat intake, create a "nutritional environment" at home that builds on your newly acquired knowledge of low-fat foods. Apply skills and strategies pertinent to other obstacles (see Steps 4 and 5), such as shopping after eating rather than when hungry, and using a list to guide selection. As you familiarize yourself with the low-fat versions of chips (e.g., baked corn or potato chips), frozen desserts (e.g., sorbet, nonfat frozen yogurt), baked goods, cereals, breads, and sauces, these should become the items with which you stock your pantry (see Section IV for details). A home environment in which only relatively low-fat food choices are available will reinforce your commitment to a reduced fat diet, until you no longer need to think about it.

It's a High-fat Jungle Out There
Your "nutritional home" will protect you from the extremes of the modern nutritional environment. One of these extremes is how much high-fat food is out there.

One key strategy is bringing food with you each day, and relying on your "food supply," rather than that provided by others. Use an insulated lunch bag, filled with some combination of fresh fruit, dried fruit, fresh vegetables, whole-grain products, and/or nonfat dairy, as an essential part of your daily routine. Set out to face the day with your handbag or valise in one hand, your snack bag in the other.

Along with the preparation of your snacks, you will need to make a commitment to avoiding the high-fat food provided by others, or simply present in your environment. The good news is, the more you reduce the fat content of your diet, the less appetizing you will tend to find fatty foods. Studies demonstrate that people initially favoring high-fat foods actually develop aversions to overly rich foods once they adjust to a low-fat diet. This is one of your goals—to develop a preference for low-fat foods.

By committing to avoid the nutritional hazards that are a part of your daily environment, and providing yourself with nutritious and low-fat snack foods, you will very readily begin to reduce your daily fat intake. By snacking regularly, you also control your appetite, leading toward more restrained and thoughtful eating throughout the day.

Don't Let "Perfect" Be the Enemy of "Good"

There are many opportunities to reduce fat content, and each is a step toward a better diet. But how many such steps you are willing to take at any given time is entirely up to you! If you feel like you are being pushed to go farther, or faster, than you want to go—slow down. You're in charge here! We're just coaching.

If you try to be "perfect" in cutting fat out of your diet, you may wind up with some foods you just don't like. And eating these may discourage you, or even cause you to give up. Don't let that happen. Progress is good; perfection is not necessary.

However committed you may be to improving your diet, and to restricting your intake of fat, you will have to admit that certain foods or dishes simply do not taste the same when the fat content is reduced. Being honest about this is essential. For eating to remain pleasurable as you pursue optimal dietary health requires that you distinguish between foods and recipes you can readily get used to, and those you can't.

If you change all of the things you can comfortably change—using the strategies above—you will dramatically reduce your fat intake. These important changes to your diet should leave plenty of room for those occasional, high-fat foods you still love, and for which there simply is no substitute. Just make sure they really are occasional! Identify your "don't mess with this!" foods, place them in the context of a prudent and healthful diet, and enjoy them thoroughly when you indulge.

Of Katz, and Kittens...

When you have five kids, what you do when your kids are born happens often enough to become tradition! With the birth of our children, Catherine and I have always celebrated—a day or two later—with our favorite dietary indulgence: fresh goat cheese, a crusty baguette, and a fine red wine.

We don't eat goat cheese often, but when we do—I sure do enjoy it! And I associate it with some of the most cherished experiences in my life.

Transitions Are Transient; Be Patient!

Once you have learned a thing or two about food labels, identified the products you like that are relatively low in fat, and gotten used to some ingredient substitutions, the hard part is over. You simply can continue buying what you are now used to buying, and eating what you are now used to eating. You have successfully met the challenge of dietary fat "addiction" when you have designed your own low-fat nutritional environment, and learned to be completely at home within its boundaries.

Obstacle/Opportunity 2: Discomfort/Inconvenience Associated with Changes to a High-Fiber Diet

The modern food supply, based largely on processed foods, tends to provide low levels of fiber. An intake of at least 25gm of fiber per day is recommended; some studies indicate additional benefits from an intake of up to 50gm per day would be better still. Yet average intake among American adults is approximately only 12gm per day. While a high-fiber intake is associated with an array of health benefits, it may also be in some ways inconvenient, increasing the volume of food you need, and potentially increasing the frequency of trips to the bathroom. Going abruptly from low-fiber intake to high-fiber intake can result in gastrointestinal discomfort. In general, any difficulty involved in adjusting to a high-fiber diet fades away pretty quickly. Putting up with the transition is worth the effort, because a high-fiber diet can help lead to reduced risk of colon cancer, to lower cholesterol, and to better weight control.

The Then/Now Conflict

To meet high energy needs with low-calorie foods, a high volume of food intake is needed. As a result, our ancestors are estimated to have consumed as much as one hundred grams of fiber per day! This is important because it suggests that we are adapted to an intake level in this range.

Many people around the world have high-fiber intakes. Dennis Burkitt, a medical missionary who spent much of his professional career in Africa, is credited with some colorful comments based on the relative fiber intake of modern and developing countries. Burkitt noted that, by world standards, the entire U.S. population is constipated!

Although we are designed for a high-fiber intake, those of us living in industrialized countries are generally not used to it. Our intestines adapt to the level of fiber in our daily diets; going from high-fiber to low-fiber intake may cause constipation, going from low intake to high may cause some discomfort.

Strategy

High fiber intake, both of soluble fiber that tends to control cholesterol, glucose, and insulin levels, and of insoluble fiber that tends to protect against colon cancer and diverticulosis, is not only a good thing in its own right, but is linked to a dietary pattern that provides many other health benefits. The same foods that are naturally high in fiber—whole grains, beans, legumes, fruits, and vegetables—are foods rich in nutrients and low in calories.

Go Slowly into That Good Diet

To get the benefits of high-fiber intake, while avoiding any potential discomfort, make gradual adjustments to your diet. You can think of this just like warming up before engaging in more vigorous activity. Gradually increase your intake of grains, fruits, and/or vegetables as you move toward better eating. If you experience bloating or discomfort, don't give up. Rather, temporarily reduce your intake of high-fiber foods to just below the level causing any discomfort, and maintain this level for roughly two weeks. Then, make another incremental increase. These slow adjustments allow the gastrointestinal system time to acclimate.

Bathe Your Fiber, Often

Drinking plenty of fluids, especially water, is important to overall health and to weight control, and can also make it easier to eat more fiber comfortably. Fluids help the gastrointestinal system to function optimally, and also perform the simple function of washing the foods we eat through the system. The recommended intake of water for an adult is about eight glasses (64 oz) a day.

Counting Beans

Many people are particularly susceptible to discomfort when eating beans or lentils. These foods have some proteins that may be difficult to digest. Here, too, gradual acclimation, with slowly increasing portions, is a fairly reliable way of avoiding problems. Because beans and lentils are nutritional powerhouses, high in protein, fiber, and many nutrients, they are a very important part of the diet. If you find that even despite gradual acclimation you have difficulty digesting these foods, the use of a commercial enzyme supplement (such as Beano), designed to break down the resistant proteins, is definitely worth trying. These products work well for most people, providing comfortable access to the health benefits of these foods.

Count Me In

Many people have no difficulty increasing fiber intake, but if you do, take your time and acclimate. Don't give up. Once you adjust to a higher intake of fiber, you, too, can gain all of the health benefits, without any discomfort.

Obstacle/Opportunity 3: Fear of Hunger

A sense of fear, or at least anxiety, associated with hunger is an important obstacle to efforts at weight control. Some people eat frequently to avoid the anxiety induced by feeling hungry, and in the process take in too many calories, and gain weight. Others, trying to avoid this very outcome, go for long periods without eating, only to binge when the time to eat finally arrives. This, too, typically leads to overindulgence, and difficulty with weight control. Whatever your strategy to control your diet and weight, you are subject, to one extent or another, to anxiety and fear provoked by hunger, and by your deep-seated desire to avoid these feelings.

The Then/Now Conflict

Starvation has been a threat to the survival of individuals, and our species, throughout all the ages. In many parts of the world, unfortunately, it still is.

For many of us, fortunate in this regard, all but the very earliest pangs of hunger are unfamiliar. True hunger, and even the early indications of its arrival, triggers a primal sense of fear. That response is built into us all as a defense against malnutrition; we are only here today at all because our ancestors avoided that threat, diligently and continuously pursuing the sense of comfort and security provided by a full belly.

Compounding the primal response to hunger is the array of signals that tend to mingle with "hunger"; much of our eating is in response to stimuli other than hunger, both social and psychological. Thus, we are driven to overeat both by hunger and the anxiety it evokes, and other cues we often mistake for hunger.

Complicating this even further, many of us, subject to weight gain, are equally anxious about eating too much. Thus, the hazards of the modern world cause us to fear eating, while the hazards of the prehistoric world cause us to fear not eating! Talk about a rock and a hard place! These competing impulses exert a strong, harmful influence on our relationship with food.

Strategy

Knowledge is not always a complete compensation for primitive drives, but it is a good start. Understand that you are naturally programmed to eat when hungry and to avoid hunger whenever possible. Trying too hard to resist this natural tendency may be swimming against the tides.

Steer Clear of Famine & Feast

The initial step in gaining control over the demands of hunger is to avoid them in a reliable, prudent way. No matter how eager you are to control your weight, we advise against going for long periods without eating. This will invariably activate the "hunger-anxiety response," primitive impulses will take over, and your control over dietary choice, and portion size, will be compromised or lost.

On the other hand, as you eat to control hunger and related anxiety, you must do so in a measured, thoughtful way. Carrots, apples, or whole-grain cereals, for example, suppress hunger as well as, or better than, pizza, muffins, candy bars, or doughnuts. What they typically do not do, however, is activate an intense and somewhat uncontrollable pleasure response. When you are eating to control hunger, you do not want to replace hunger with another stimulus that is just as difficult to control!

Take Control, Choose Wisely

Therefore, you should eat regularly, whenever you begin to feel hungry. But you cannot allow the nutritional environment to determine your choices. Develop a system, whether you spend your days at home, in the car, or in an office, that allows you to control your own food supply. A simple approach is to pack an insulated snack bag every day. The arrangement you need to make with yourself every day is this: 1) I will have food at hand to eat whenever I get hungry, so I don't need to worry about "starving" or feeling deprived, but 2) I will eat only those foods I bring with me for this very purpose. Choose foods that are nutritious, low in calories, and filling. Have them handy, and eat them often, as a way of controlling the primal fear of hunger.

Healthy Momentum

At first, you may work hard to eat the "proper" snack foods, and will still be tempted by fast foods, doughnuts, pizza, and such. But before long, the idea that you eat what you prepare will become second nature.

Your ability to select foods for your snack pack (see Section IV) will improve with time, until this becomes just a habit. But this is just the beginning. The space taken up by these nutritious foods will leave less room for higher-calorie, less nutritious foods. Simply by addressing the fear of hunger in a productive way, you will start, little by little, to shift the entire pattern of your diet from high-calorie, low-nutrient foods that threaten your health and waistline, to foods rich in nutrients and relatively low in calories, that enhance both!

Simplify

As this trend takes hold, you will find your relationship with food simplifying. Knowing you can eat whenever you get hungry, and be increasingly confident about how to do so in a healthful way, you will no longer be tempted to avoid food. The fear of hunger, and the fear of food (in excess) will tend to fade together. Removing both the "rock" and the "hard place" that have previously bounded your efforts to eat well, you suddenly have room to maneuver. The primal fear of hunger, and the modern fear of getting fat, can be mastered!

Obstacle/Opportunity 4: Innate Preference for Sugar

There is clear evidence from scientific studies in both animals and humans that a preference for sweet-tasting food is innate. That is to say, we like sugar even before we are born! Then, the more exposure we have to sugar, the more we like it.

While sugar is not clearly linked to weight-control problems per se, it is considered a "vehicle" for dietary fat. In other words, sugary foods are often high-fat, calorie-dense foods as well; the pleasant taste of sugar stimulates high intake, while the fat does much of the damage in terms of calories, weight gain, and adverse health effects.

Compounding all of this even further, the satiety threshold for sweet in the brain is higher than for other tastes. This means that we need to eat more sugar to get full than we do of other types of food. This makes sugar particularly irresistible.

Sugar is everywhere in the modern, highly processed diet. Even in "salty" foods not thought of as sweet, such as ketchup, mustard, relishes, chips, breads, or crackers, sugar is often a prominent ingredient, stimulating our taste buds even when we don't know it's there!

The Then/Now Conflict

For our ancestors, sugar was a quick source of energy, and the foods it was found in (fruit, honey, and plants such as sugar cane) were safe. In nature, bitter foods are often toxic, while sweet foods are rarely so.

So the tendency to like sweet was handed down from generation to generation until it became an indelible part of us, built into our genetic code. A "sweet tooth" is not a matter of willpower, it's a matter of gene power!

With this strong "demand" and an abundant supply, consumption of sugar in the modern diet is high. Simple sugar in the diet is associated with tooth decay, increased insulin release, and increased consumption of fat and calories, among other possible adverse effects.

Strategy: Put Sugar in Its Place

First, make some general commitment about the acceptable place of sweet foods in your diet. For example, you might take an extreme position and ban dessert altogether, or you might limit it to one meal a day, or a certain number of meals per week. Such a commitment is only as good as your follow-through, of course. But making decisions about tempting foods at a time other than when you are tempted is a good strategy in general. If you are uncertain about your ability to comply with the plan, you might want to share the pledge with a friend and engage their support.

Once you have decided when sweets are acceptable, define carefully the foods that you want to consider "sweets." Fresh and dried fruit, for example, while concentrated sources of natural sugars, shouldn't count because they are nutrient and fiber dense. The foods to avoid are those that are processed, offering lots of sugar and calories without nutrients and fiber along with sugary soft drinks (see Section IV for more guidance).

Expect the Unexpected Sugar...

You will then need to read food labels to find the sugar you expect, as well as the sugar you do not. Names that indicate the addition of sweetener include: sucrose, fructose, corn syrup, etc. The first goal is to recognize where sugar is finding its way into your diet, so you can make adjustments to limit your intake. The second goal is to identify those sweet foods that are also providing a hefty dose of fat and calories. In efforts to control weight and improve dietary health, these foods are best avoided altogether.

Sweet Substitutions

To indulge a desire for sweet, but avoid the fat and calories that tend to come along for the ride, you should identify foods that satisfy the need for sweet at a low dose of fat and calories. A good example is sorbet (or other nonfat frozen dessert) as a substitute for ice cream. Both provide sugar, and neither could be considered a "health" food. But we have already taken the position that eating should be fun as well as healthful, and we don't intend to abandon that position now! The goal here is to preserve the pleasure, and minimize the cost.

While you might prefer, for example, chocolate ice cream to chocolate sorbet, that preference can be overcome. First, we tend to prefer the familiar to the unfamiliar. But the unfamiliar can be made familiar by trying it, and sticking with it for a while.

Further, a preference is sometimes only apparent with a direct comparison. So, in a side-by-side taste test, you might pick ice cream over sorbet (you might not, if used to the sorbet). That is quite different from craving a sweet, cold refreshing dessert on a hot summer night, opening your freezer and finding nothing but sorbet. No side-by-side comparison, just the more prudent choice. It will satisfy you. Giving up the fat to preserve the pleasure of sweet is a modest price to pay to have your proverbial "cake" (sorbet, actually) and eat it, too!

Of Sugar & Science

Another strategy for reducing sugar intake is to make use of artificial sweeteners. These, for the most part, are likely to be safe if eaten in moderate quantities, and most offer clear advantages for dental health. Another potential advantage of artificial sweeteners is that they do not elicit a release of insulin. However, if combined with excess fat in processed foods, artificial sweeteners can promote excess intake as readily as natural sugars, so this strategy should be applied with caution. It is probably of greatest utility to apply this strategy to soft drinks, which in general do not provide fat, but can provide many empty calories from sugar.

How to Behave When Sweet's What You Crave

Another issue with sweets is that they may induce strong cravings. A craving for chocolate, for example, has been detected in human populations from time to time! In general, the best approach to a strong craving for a sweet (or almost any food) is to indulge it. Go right to the heart of the craving, but control the "damage" by eating a modest portion of whatever is calling your name.

Learning to Love the Food You're With

Finally, and perhaps most importantly, the overall pattern of your diet strongly shapes your preferences and tendencies. Even though you were born to like sugar, if your diet shifts, step-by-step, to one richer in nutrient-dense, calorie-dilute, natural foods, there will simply be less place for processed sugar in your diet. With these gains, do forgive yourself for any occasional indulgence; after all, it's perfectly natural!

Obstacle/Opportunity 5
Persistent Appetite (Leptin Resistance)

You may never have heard of leptin, let alone resistance to it. That's just the point! How could you hope to overcome this challenge to eating well without knowing there even was such a thing?!

While there are many genes that influence weight control, the "Ob gene" is thus far considered one of the more important. This gene is responsible for the production of a protein called leptin. Leptin is produced by fat cells, or adipocytes.

Ordinarily, fat cells that are satisfied with their supply of energy release leptin to signal to the brain that they are "full." In some people, the brain cells that should respond to leptin are insensitive, or resistant, to the message. As a result, appetite stays turned on long after it should be shut off. This leads to overeating, which naturally leads to weight gain. Weight gain in turn may make leptin resistance more severe.

The Stark-Raving Craving...

Wednesday evening, 8:30 P.M., about one-and-one-half hours after dinner, and for no apparent reason, Jenna had a craving for ice cream. And she'd already had dessert! So, she thought, I'll have something healthier instead. She ate a few raisins, but still had the craving. She ate a slice of bread with jam, but still had the craving. She munched on a few crackers, but still had the craving. She...ate the ice cream! At least the craving went away...

Our advice: keep sorbet or nonfat frozen yogurt in the house, instead of ice cream, and if that's what you crave, go right to it! Jenna now does—and it works!

The Then/Now Conflict

For our ancestors, the importance of fat tissue reserves as defense against famine required that the fat reserves in the body have some means to indicate whether they were full, empty, or in between—a Stone Age "fuel gauge," if you will. While the details of the biochemical signaling related to appetite and satiety are intricate, and not fully worked out, the important role of leptin is clear. Leptin is released from adipose tissue stores when they are full, binds to cells in the brain, and blocks the release of another body chemical, neuropeptide Y, that promotes appetite. Thus, high levels of leptin shut off appetite.

When leptin levels fall, as happens when fat tissue reserves start to dwindle, neuropeptide Y levels rise again, and with them goes appetite. All of this served our ancestors well by helping to ensure an energy reserve.

Obesity, a state quite new for our species, is often associated with high levels of leptin. While the reasons for this are uncertain, one possibility is that a relative insensitivity to leptin may predispose to weight gain by leaving appetite stimulated long after it should shut down. Another possibility is that excessive numbers of fat cells place excessive demands on the appetite centers in the brain, and just as a daycare worker grows tolerant to the chatter of many children, the centers grow tolerant to the persistent demands of leptin, eventually tuning them out.

Whatever the explanation or explanations for this state, an appetite that tends to remain stimulated when it should be suppressed obviously represents a considerable challenge to weight-control efforts.

Strategy: Get in Touch with Your Appetite

One of the principal difficulties in attempting to lose or even control weight is the tendency to be hungry. Any diet that can be used over the course of a lifetime to control weight must satisfy the appetite.

Fortunately, the health-promoting dietary pattern recommended throughout this book has many features that make it ideal for controlling both weight and appetite. Snacking regularly allows for continuous signals to the brain that food energy is being provided. This helps to reduce appetite signals, even if there is some degree of leptin resistance at work.

Eating foods in the categories especially recommended—grains, fruits, vegetables—results in a diet that is high in volume and fiber, nutritious, low in calories, yet filling. There is some evidence to suggest that soluble fiber may be especially good at making you feel full, providing another benefit of high intake of grains, beans, lentils, vegetables, and fruits.

Putting Protein to Work

There is, as well, some evidence that protein is the most filling, or *satiating* of the macronutrient classes. If this is so, then a protein intake toward the higher end of the recommended range, approximately 20 percent of calories, may be helpful to those who always feel hungry. Higher protein intake than this cannot be recommended, because it is not consistent with the overall evidence for health promotion.

Fat, the most calorie-dense macronutrient class, has, in general, a low *satiety index*, a measure of a food's capacity to induce a feeling of fullness. Thus, leptin resistance is one reason among all of the others mentioned elsewhere for restricting intake of dietary fat.

By snacking on appropriate foods often, restricting fat intake, consuming appropriate amounts of protein from sources not rich in fat, and eating plenty of unprocessed plant foods rich in soluble fiber, the challenge of leptin resistance can be successfully met.

Obstacle/Opportunity 6
Thrifty Metabolism (Insulin Resistance)

We are, as a species, designed to be fuel-efficient by necessity. Insulin plays a fundamental role in the storage and utilization of food energy, and is thus an important regulator of our energy-efficiency. The brisk release of insulin when food is ingested helps to ensure that none of the energy in food goes to waste, that all of it is either used immediately for the work of muscle or other tissues, or is stored.

This same mechanism may contribute to weight gain, obesity, and the development of diabetes when food is abundantly available all of the time. The brisk insulin release that is appropriate when food is intermittent becomes a liability when its supply is constant.

The Then/Now Conflict

In many ways, insulin can be thought of as an energy sponge, its release following a meal helping to ensure that every available calorie is put to good use. Glucose, the simple sugar we use as a preferred fuel, enters many tissues, including muscle, guided by insulin.

But insulin does much more. It promotes the storage of excess glucose as glycogen, a carbohydrate energy depot. When the relatively modest storage capacity for glycogen has been reached, insulin causes carbohydrate, and even protein, to be converted into triglycerides for storage in fat tissue. A lean adult weighing 154 lbs (70 kg) has roughly 1,200 kcal stored in glycogen, and 100 times as much, or 120,000 kcal stored in adipose tissue.

The calories stored in glycogen are enough to survive only twelve to eighteen hours of fasting. Thus, our ancestors were very dependent on their ability to store calories as fat to survive any sustained period of deprivation. Those that tended to release insulin briskly following a meal were also those most likely to produce triglycerides, and store enough energy in fat cells to see them through the hard times.

Over the eons, with each recurrent cycle of feast and famine, those prehistoric humans that were metabolically efficient survived, and reproduced; those that were less so did not. We thus became more and more the offspring of metabolically efficient people, until this was a fundamental characteristic of our species.

In modern context, this characteristic has been converted from asset to liability. Food energy is available to us in constant abundance. Energy efficiency is not necessary under such conditions. In fact, those individuals who are least energy efficient, those that can eat "whatever they want" and not gain weight, are often envied in our society. While they are the most resistant to obesity in modern context, these individuals would have been most vulnerable to starvation had they lived among our ancestors. Advantage, or disadvantage, is determined by context.

Most of us release insulin briskly when we eat. Because we eat often, tend to eat more than we need, and because often our food is highly processed, low in fiber, and high in simple sugars and fat, our release of insulin in any twenty-four-hour period is high.

Constant, high levels of insulin release likely cause the insulin receptor to become somewhat resistant to the message insulin delivers. High levels of insulin also contribute to weight gain, which increases insulin requirements, causing insulin levels to rise even higher. This, in turn, may contribute to even further receptor resistance.

Eventually, this tremendous demand causes the cells in the pancreas that make insulin to wear out. When this occurs, type II (non-insulin dependent) *diabetes mellitus* develops.

The susceptibility to insulin resistance, weight gain, and diabetes that comes from combining Stone Age traits, tendencies, and genes with the modern environment does not affect all of us to the same degree. Just as we differ from one another in height, eye color, skin tone, speed, strength, or dexterity, so, too, do we differ in our metabolic efficiency. Some people and ethnic groups are very much influenced by metabolic efficiency and insulin resistance, others much less so. But as a species, overall, metabolic efficiency is a potentially important obstacle to weight control.

If you gain weight easily, you are probably metabolically "thrifty." If you gain weight mostly around the middle, have high triglycerides, high blood pressure, and/or low HDL cholesterol, you may well be insulin resistant.

Strategy

An understanding of the links between our prehistoric design, metabolic efficiency, and insulin resistance is the first step in meeting the challenge of this condition, and exploiting the opportunity it affords. Avoid thinking of metabolic efficiency as bad luck, or the product of bad or defective genes. Rather, accept this is part of who and what we are, part of what we needed to be throughout all of our evolutionary history.

Driving a Fuel-efficient Metabolism

Fuel-efficiency requires moderation in the supply of fuel. Our energy-efficiency also helps to explain why regular physical activity is so important. We were designed both to go a long way, and to do so on relatively limited fuel. Our health is enhanced if we can approximate the conditions for which we are adapted and designed.

The Art of Grazing

A specific strategy for the control of insulin release is to snack regularly on appropriate foods. There is some evidence to suggest that if the same number of calories is spread out in multiple small meals rather than several large ones, insulin release is reduced.

Make Friends with Fiber

Soluble, or *viscous* fiber is a category of indigestible plant material that includes, among others, guar gum, psyllium, pectin, and ß-glucan, and is abundant in oats and other grains, apples, berries, beans, and lentils. As opposed to insoluble fiber, soluble fiber dissolves in water. In the intestines, soluble fiber slows down the absorption into the blood stream of both fat molecules and glucose, lowering the amount of insulin needed to metabolize a meal.

In addition, soluble fiber takes up space without providing any calories, and thus makes foods more filling and satisfying. This is true of insoluble fiber, or roughage, as well. Insoluble fiber is especially abundant in whole grains such as wheat, and in many vegetables.

Consider the Glycemic Index

A property of foods whose importance to insulin metabolism should be considered, but not exaggerated, is the *glycemic index* (GI). The GI is a measure of how much a food raises blood glucose (and, consequently, insulin) relative to a slice of white bread, which is used as the reference standard. The bread is set at a GI of 100; a GI less than 100 means a lesser tendency to raise blood sugar than the bread, and higher than 100 means a greater tendency (see Section IV for more details). The GI serves as one basis for the "exchange lists" used in the dietary management of diabetes.

The usefulness of the GI is limited, however. First, the GI pertains only to single foods. We tend to eat foods in combinations, and when we do, the properties of one food influence another. A food high in soluble fiber, for example, eaten together with a high GI food, will prevent any abrupt rise in blood glucose, or insulin. High fiber foods will in fact modify glycemic responses to other foods eaten even hours later. Second, individual responses to even single foods vary considerably. What raises your blood sugar a lot may raise ours just a little, and vice versa.

Another factor limiting the usefulness of the GI is that it is not a reliable guide toward health-promoting foods, or away from foods of limited nutritional value. Ice cream has a much lower GI than white bread, while carrots have a much higher GI. The interpretation that one should eat ice cream, but avoid carrots to control weight or promote health would be, of course, ridiculous!

Thus, use the GI, if you use it at all, only as a general guide to help you select the more complex carbohydrate foods from among those in any given category, such as breads, cereals, or desserts. We recommend against using it as a means of deciding what dietary pattern makes sense. If you have diabetes, the GI takes on slightly more importance, but even then, your overall dietary pattern is far more important than the GI of any given food.

Let a Little of the Mediterranean into Your Diet

There are studies to suggest that insulin release can be improved by monounsaturated fat, such as is found in olive oil. There does not appear to be any evidence that diets high in monounsaturated fat are superior to diets high in fiber in controlling insulin, however. Prudence suggests that the benefits of both of these strategies be combined.

While monounsaturated fat offers health benefits not found in saturated or trans fat, it of course has the same energy density (9kcal/gm), and thus could contribute to weight gain if not consumed in moderation. A high-fiber diet can help achieve that moderation.

No News Is Good News

So, when all of the strategies for controlling insulin release are considered, they add up to the same diet recommended for health in general! So there's no real "news" here, and that's the best news of all. The same basic strategies come together to help you over a wide array of obstacles.

In attempting to manage insulin release and metabolic efficiency, you can, and should, rely on the same dietary pattern advisable for every other goal of nutritional health. A diet abundant in grains, vegetables, and fruits is nutritious, low in calories, and high in fiber. Add regular physical activity, which is important for weight regulation, and which lowers insulin requirements by conditioning muscle tissue, and you have an excellent recipe for insulin control.

No One Can Eat Just One—Meals, and Insulin Requirements. While processed carbohydrate may raise glucose and insulin more than fat on a "per-meal" basis in the short term, fat in the diet tends to lead to weight gain, and ultimately it is weight gain that affects insulin levels most. Complex carbohydrate is associated both with weight control in the long-term, and with a relatively low release of insulin in the short-term.

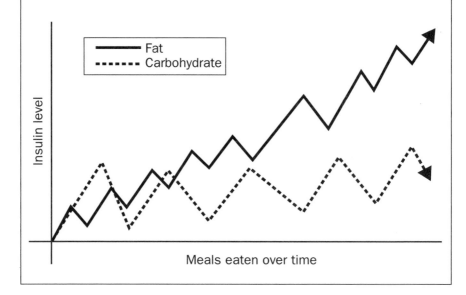

Obstacle/Opportunity 7
Normal/Natural Tendency to Binge Eat

While there is a bona fide eating disorder known as "binge-eating disorder," most of us have this tendency to one degree or another. Ask yourself, for example, whether you've ever overeaten and regretted it. If so, you've binged; join the club! When tempting and appetizing food is constantly available in both abundance and variety, the tendency to binge, even if partially controlled, can lead to serious difficulty with weight control.

The Then/Now Conflict

Just as the lean, gaunt lion on a nature program makes a kill and soon after is seen with a belly that drags on the ground, all we know suggests that our ancestors were binge eaters whenever they could be. The next meal was uncertain; the meal at hand was quite appropriately devoured for all it was worth!

The tendency to eat heartily, and indeed to overeat, when food is readily available, is age-old, seen throughout the animal kingdom, and both normal and rational. By understanding the tendency and its modern context, and taking some simple protective steps, the risk of overindulgence can be controlled.

Note that our ancestors did not possess a self-discipline we lack. They simply lacked the food supply we possess.

Strategy

If you overeat, and occasionally you almost certainly will, and blame yourself for lack of restraint you add, in the most literal sense, insult to injury.

Don't Beat Yourself Up

Our advice—our fervent request to you—is to recall that you were designed to binge. Doing so has regrettable consequences when you are struggling to control your weight, especially when one binge follows another. But it says nothing about a flaw in your character. You are being driven by four million years of evolution: a powerful engine, indeed.

If, and when, you lapse, therefore, be understanding and forgiving. This is essential to your ability to confront the challenging obstacles of the modern nutritional environment. Add to the challenges of this environment the unnecessary weight of self-reproach, embarrassment, or remorse and you simply have too much to carry. Set the burden down. If overeating has been undermining your will and self-esteem, it's time to acknowledge that you were simply behaving the way normal humans behave when food is accessible.

Control Hunger

Controlling the inclination to binge begins with the avoidance of hunger. Many people trying to control their weight avoid food for long stretches, typically during the workday. But avoiding food for hours on end almost invariably results not only in calorie overcompensation at day's end, but reactivating our primal fear of hunger. Whatever your commitment to restraint, when you give in to hunger after resisting it for hours, its powerful influence is likely to overwhelm you. There are other reasons for avoiding long periods without eating. There is some evidence that eating even the same number of calories in intermittent, large meals, results in more insulin release than those calories distributed in more frequent, smaller meals, as shown below.

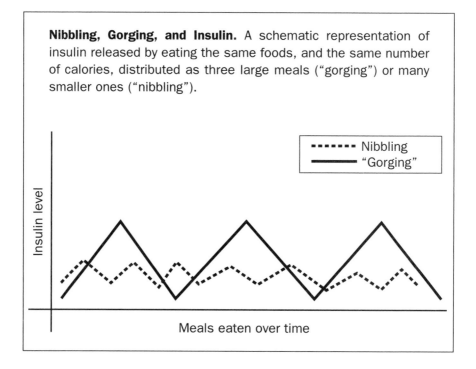

Nibbling, Gorging, and Insulin. A schematic representation of insulin released by eating the same foods, and the same number of calories, distributed as three large meals ("gorging") or many smaller ones ("nibbling").

- - - - - - Nibbling
———— "Gorging"

Insulin level

Meals eaten over time

By avoiding food, then giving in, we add the power of insulin to produce fat to the powerful fear of hunger that compels us to overeat.

Beware of Food Fights

Another noteworthy disadvantage of avoiding food for extended periods is that it complicates further an already tense and complicated relationship. You may think about food, and/or your health, weight, or appearance almost constantly. Food is perhaps at once your constant friend, and your most troublesome challenge. Could a relationship be much more complicated than that?

Spoil Your Appetite

Become comfortable with the notion that you are not subject to true hunger, let alone starvation. To do this, you should have food readily available all the time. You must, in fact, follow the advice your mother never intended to give, and "spoil" your appetite by snacking.

The exact approach that's right for you will depend on where, when, and how you work, whether in the home or out, day or night, alone or with company. Assuming, for the moment, you work in an office with coworkers during the day, here are some simple steps to take.

First, purchase an insulated "lunch" bag. The surest way to survive in a toxic nutritional environment is to create your own environment, and take it with you. This concept is not foreign. You dress for the weather each day, light clothes in summer, warm in winter. Imagine going out with no concept of the season, let alone the forecast. You might find yourself in shorts in a snowstorm, in heavy wool when it's one hundred degrees and humid. Going out into the "nutritional" environment and hoping for the best is just about as promising, and prudent.

Your lunch bag (a snack bag, really) should be filled each day with foods you like, but not foods you like too much. Intensely pleasurable foods, such as, for example, candy bars, are generally calorie-dense, nutrient-poor, and very difficult to control.

To use snacking as a curb on appetite and a means of simplifying your relationship with diet requires thoughtful choices. Such choices are convenient to pack up, nutritious, low in calories, simple, and satisfying. Good choices for snack foods include fresh fruit, fresh vegetables, dried fruit, whole-grain cereals, whole-grain breads (without spreads), whole-grain crackers (with no added oil/fat), and nonfat dairy. These foods, kept close at hand, are your first and best defense against hunger during the day.

Food is often eaten for reasons other than hunger, such as stress, boredom, or a need for gratification; healthy snacks are your defense against these vulnerabilities as well. If you go all day without eating, even if you don't feel you are resisting hunger, you are missing the relief of stress that chewing on something satisfying can provide. That unresolved stress likely contributes to an unrestrained binge at the end of the day. Snack well throughout the day, and you won't carry that stress home with you.

Get Going

As already mentioned, unless you have a truly exceptional work environment (or home), you likely experience some stress most days. We tend to convert that stress into something like hunger, and it contributes to the tendency to overindulge. Physical activity is one of the very best ways to alleviate stress.

But leaving time for physical activity at the end of the day is particularly unpleasant if you are "starving," as you might well be if you avoided food all day. A well-chosen snack in the mid to late afternoon can blunt appetite enough to allow for after-work/end-of-day exercise, which in turn will burn calories, alleviate stress, and generally control appetite further. A winning combination if ever there was one! The health advantages of consistent physical activity are considerable, and weight control over time is nearly impossible unless physical activity is part of the formula.

By "venting" with exertion at the end of the day, you will likely not only burn some calories, but also take in fewer. Dinner tends to be more thoughtful following some exercise. Insulin levels tend to stay lower. The benefits go on and on.

Create Your Own "Safe" Nutritional Environment

As you begin to create your own protective nutritional environment, you must consider it is little more than an oasis in a vast and oppressive desert. Just beyond your snack bag, other choices are likely to beckon: food brought to work by well-meaning coworkers, a vending machine, a restaurant, or cafeteria.

Consider a "pact" to yourself or someone else to guard against the many temptations of the nutritional environment. Vow, for a month, or two, then three, then longer, to eat only the foods you bring to work. You can expand this to foods you purchase by deciding in advance what the acceptable options are. For example, you may vary your routine by purchasing a salad or sandwich, but you shouldn't open the choices to anything at all. The pizza and doughnuts to be found in so many office environments are tempting and tasty, but calorically dense and threatening to your waistline and health. Rather than trying to resist temptation when experiencing it, which is very difficult, resist it in advance when it's easier to do. *"I will not eat food brought to the office for the next two months…"* simplifies your decisions and helps to keep you safe.

And remember, snacking is no protection against overeating if snacking becomes overeating. The same powerful forces that can lead to harmful binges at day's end can do the same all day long if not appropriately controlled.

Call in the Cavalry

Closely related to the issue of resisting the tempting foods you will encounter is the appropriateness of asking for help. If you are overweight, you are, forgive us for saying so, not the only one who knows it! It's apparent. If instead of your weight you are trying to improve a less visible health risk through diet, your friends would likely help you if they knew about it.

Either way, ask for help. You are not "dieting," and need not be embarrassed. You are trying to improve your diet, your weight, your health—an issue that will resonate with most of the people you tell. So tell. Ask your friends, family, and coworkers to help you. Let them know, in advance, that improving your diet will be tough enough with help, too tough if they try to lead you astray. Ask not to be tempted with foods you are trying to avoid. This strategy is obviously simple, and extremely helpful, but largely overlooked. With a well-provisioned snack bag, and supportive friends, you are well on your way.

Kevin's Friends...

Kevin had been a high-school football star, and remained very athletic through college. So the idea that at forty-two he was fat and out-of-shape was hard for him to take. He could barely admit it to himself, let alone anyone else.

Se he tried to get his weight under control on the sly, not telling his buddies what he was doing. So, of course, they continued to offer the usual—pizza, chips, chicken wings, beer. Feeling embarrassed to say no, Kevin would generally go along. When he did try to resist, his buddies would tease him, and he would give in then. His weight was going nowhere but up.

We suggested he let his buddies in on his "secret." As it happened, Mark and Steve were just as eager to drop a few pounds as Kevin. They worked together to change some of their eating habits, and have lost twenty-one pounds—as a group effort! They've also added basketball two nights a week to their routine. The whole group is thinner, fitter, and happier.

Friends in need...friends, indeed!

Address Your Settings

While the portable snack-pack, kept in a desk drawer, car, or anywhere close at hand, may provide some protection against the nutritional environment outside the home, it will provide little protection against such an environment under your own roof. You, alone or with other household members, control the nutritional environment in your own home. Make it a safe one.

You will almost certainly want something sweet, or salty, or crunchy on occasion. The time to decide whether to satisfy, for example, an inclination for sweet with ice cream, or fat-free sorbet, is not when the inclination asserts itself, but before.

If the ice cream is not to be found in your freezer, and the sorbet is, your choice is straightforward, and your sweet tooth will be satisfied without the density of fat and calories that ice cream provides. This approach, by the way, is also appropriate for cultivating healthful eating habits in children, a common challenge for parents. You can safeguard against our natural tendency to binge both by using strategies that help you avoid bingeing, and strategies that prevent harm if you do binge. When confronting the challenge of four million years of natural selection, better two lines of defense than one!

Anticipate the Sirens' Song on Your Nutritional Odyssey

You have probably heard before now that you should not shop when hungry; we add our support to this wise and simple adage. Eat a snack (a prudent one) before you shop, or if pressed for time, while on your way. Whenever possible, make a shopping list in advance, and do so after eating, not before.

These strategies can be placed in a historical context millenia old. In *The Odyssey* by Homer, Odysseus (Ulysses) had himself bound to his ship's mast to resist the call of the Sirens, knowing he could not resist it otherwise. Before being tempted, he took precautions that saved him when a compelling and dangerous temptation was encountered.

On the nutritional Odyssey the modern environment requires of us all, similar precautions are needed. None of us is simply strong enough to resist the siren song of so many luscious and tempting foods calling out to us. But by knowing where and when to expect such temptation, and taking precautions in advance, we, like Odysseus, can come safely home. Lashed tightly to your list, your resolve, your knowledge, and your post-snack satiety, you can pass safely among the temptations of the supermarket.

Beware the Buffet!

Temptation is particularly strong under certain circumstances. Buffets not only potently activate our tendency to overindulge, they also play to a particular vulnerability, called sensory specific satiety. Briefly, sensory specific satiety is our tendency to remain hungry longer, and eat more, when a greater variety of foods and flavors is available.

The simplest, and safest strategy regarding buffets if you are striving to control and improve your diet is: avoid them. If they are an inescapable part of your routine, make them so as seldom as possible.

If you can't do even that, rely on prudent snacking just prior. Decide in advance, not once tempted, what foods, and how many, will be acceptable. Stick to these decisions either through a commitment to yourself, or as discussed above, with the help and support of others. The sequence of your selections at buffets can also be important. Start rather than end with salad. Avoid concentrated sources of fat and calories, such as processed meats and cheeses, altogether or at least until already somewhat full.

And, of course, if you do attend the occasional buffet, and do, despite both good intentions and strategies, overindulge, forgive yourself and resume your prior efforts. There is no cause for remorse in perfectly normal human behavior. You are not particularly good at flying, breathing under water, or running on all fours, either, if you need to consider other comparably unreasonable reasons to beat up on yourself! Give yourself a break, and get back to your good intentions.

Holiday Cheer, and Peer Pressure

The strategies useful for buffets also help to meet the challenges of social gatherings and holidays. When reasonable, snack in advance. Eat the low-calorie, nutritious foods, such as salad, first. Identify, in advance rather than when tempted, what if any foods you will particularly avoid. Decide, in advance, how many, and what size, servings of different dishes you will take.

And enlist help. Social gatherings are nearly impossible to contend with if you attempt dietary restraint on the sly. Tell everyone; there is no reason to be ashamed, or discrete. Recall that a majority of American adults are overweight; your struggle is everyone's struggle. If you ask for help, you may get it, and the very occasions that most tended to undermine your resolve may now provide valuable social support. Your commitment to dietary health may even be contagious, spreading health benefits to friends and loved ones who join in your efforts.

When You Can't Beat 'Em...

A final and particular challenge in efforts not to binge is a craving. Cravings are sudden, strong desires to eat a particular food or flavor. We recommend three strategies for dealing with cravings.

First, as discussed above, create a nutritional environment at work and home that controls the available options. Second, make a particular effort to have the optimal version of foods you tend to crave available (e.g., oil-free baked chips; nonfat frozen yogurt, etc; see Section IV). And third, give in swiftly!

Consider the times you've tried to resist a craving by making other food choices, one after another, until you finally gave in to the craving as well. Get right to the point. Eat the food that will satisfy the craving, and move on. Unless you have unusually frequent or compelling cravings, this simple approach will serve you well.

You Can't Win 'Em All

Even a perfect line of defense is occasionally breached by a powerful counterforce. The modern nutritional environment is a powerful counterforce indeed, to both strategy and resolve. It may occasionally lead you to binge, no matter how good your strategies.

However, all you need to do to get the benefits of eating well is succeed most of the time. Diet should be an everyday source of pleasure, just not excessive, uncontrollable, and harmful pleasure. And if on occasion you feast, enjoy it! In all honesty, I eat myself very nearly sick every Thanksgiving, and don't regret a forkful!

Use particular restraint and commitment while getting used to a new way of eating. Once a prudent diet becomes familiar and easy, you can safely let loose from time to time. If getting pleasure from food, and also getting pleasure from a prudent diet that provides you with control of your weight and promotion of your health, is "having your cake and eating it, too," then it can be done. *Bon appetit!*

Obstacle/Opportunity 8
Normal Preference for Familiar Foods

There is a strong human tendency to like the familiar, and it has a considerable influence on what we like to eat. Consider how diverse diets are around the globe. Our taste buds can adapt to anything from fried ants to *foie gras*, endive to eels. Yet you are likely very cautious if ever something completely unfamiliar winds up on your plate.

But because we all have common genetic origins, differences in cultural eating patterns and taste preference have nothing to do with differences in our taste buds. Rather, we learn to like eating what we get used to eating.

Children perhaps best display the reluctance we all can feel toward new and untried food.

Parent: *"Try this, it's good."*

Child: *"But I don't like it."*

Parent: *"How can you not like it; you've never even tried it?"*

Child: *"Yeah...but I don't like it!"*

This strong preference for the familiar, and a reluctance to eat the unfamiliar, is of course a considerable obstacle to eating well when the familiar diet is high in fat, salt, sugar, and calories, and low in nutrients and fiber.

The Then/Now Conflict

During most of human history, the bulk of our ancestors' food came from gathering, and what they found to eat varied by location. They were thus continuously challenged with the absolute necessity of trying new and unfamiliar foods in order to survive, coupled with the very real risk that any new food tried might be lethal! Anthropologists refer to the dilemma our ancestors faced as *the omnivore's paradox*. There are actually four million years of evolutionary history supporting the child that says, "I don't like it!" without ever having tried it!

In the prehistoric world, the more a food looked and tasted like foods known to be safe, the less risky it was apt to be. The more unfamiliar a food, the more threatening. Under these circumstances, natural selection would tend to favor individuals who were willing to try new foods when threatened with starvation, but who stuck with the familiar whenever possible.

Strategy

The strong influence of familiarity on dietary selection makes change difficult.

Anticipate that making any dietary changes will require a transition period. The change to a health-promoting dietary pattern is certainly worthwhile, but getting there requires commitment. However, the effort involved is relatively short-lived.

Making New (Food) Friends

You have likely heard the optimistic expression "a stranger is simply a friend you haven't yet met." This applies fairly well to untried foods, too.

Once tried, foods are no longer unfamiliar. And the longer you stick with a new food, or dish, recipe or meal, or even a new dietary pattern, the more familiar it becomes. The very force that made converting to it challenging, starts to make continuing with it easy!

This process is not wishful thinking, but is well supported by scientific evidence. In the *Iowa Women's Health Trial*, for example, women assigned to a low-fat diet found it difficult at first. However, a year after the trial, the women who had adapted to eating low-fat foods not only preferred such foods, but actually had a distaste for many of the high-fat foods they used to prefer! Taste is malleable, and you can guide it toward a particular dietary pattern just as effectively as it tends to guide you. Time to take charge!

A simple experiment you can conduct in a week or two may help you deal successfully with the challenge of dietary familiarity. Pick one high-fat, or highly processed food you eat, and identify a lower fat, or more nutritious substitute. Veggie burgers for hamburgers might work, baked corn chips for fried, nonfat granola for regular, chocolate sorbet for chocolate ice cream. There are many options, but the experiment depends on a one-for-one food substitution.

Using milk as an example, most people who drink whole or 2 percent milk find skim milk too watery. But this is really just the power of the familiar. Switch to skim milk with a commitment to use only skim milk for two weeks. If you're like most people, by the end of two weeks, you will have acclimated fully to skim milk, and whole milk may actually seem too rich, and unappetizing. You have just made a dietary change that can reduce your intake of fat and calories; you're on your way!

Opportunity for such substitutions is one of the advantages of the variety the modern food supply makes available. A number of dairies produce fat-free milk fortified with milk proteins so that the taste and texture is more like that of whole milk, or 2 percent milk. These products, and others like them, ease the transition to more healthful eating.

Slow and Steady Wins the Race

An often helpful consideration in making new foods familiar is to go slowly. Keep in mind that any additions, deletions, or substitutions— *any*—that make your diet more health-promoting are a good achievement, and success. You might well benefit from a complete "dietary overhaul," but you will obtain some portion of that benefit with each small change for the better you make in your diet. Some may prefer a "cold turkey" approach, changing everything at once. But you will likely take some comfort in knowing that slow, food by food, dish by dish progress is still progress, and a very legitimate approach to a healthful way of eating.

Taking small and gradual steps along the way to eating well is useful because it allows the overall diet to remain familiar, even as individual foods are changed. Another way of achieving the same thing is to change the nutrient profile of your food, while keeping the basic taste and appearance familiar. Your favorite chicken, meat, vegetable, or fish dishes; soups or stews; sauces, spreads, and dressing, can almost always be prepared with more healthful ingredients. The specifics—cooking, shopping, recipe recommendations, and ingredient substitutions—are provided in Section IV.

Putting the Power of the Familiar to Work for You

Each food you change in your diet makes the overall composition of your diet change slightly. As the fat, or salt, or sugar content of your diet comes down slightly, you acclimate to this lower intake level: it becomes familiar. As the new pattern becomes the familiar, and preferred pattern, the effort involved in maintaining it disappears; it becomes, simply, your way of eating. This provides an opportunity to make another small change, and another, and another. Once you have adopted, and gotten used to, a health-promoting dietary pattern, the power of the familiar becomes your ally, making it easy to maintain a diet that will promote your health and weight control, forever.

Obstacle/Opportunity 9
Normal/Natural Preference for Salt

A preference for salt is, if not innate in humans, very easily acquired. The addition of salt to the modern food supply tends to make food tastier and more palatable, and to increase our preference for salt, which in turn increases our salt intake further. The results are a high intake of salt, and the stimulation of our appetite by salt that leads to increased intake of sugar, fat, and calories, too.

The Then/Now Conflict

Salt, or sodium, in nature is relatively scarce. Animal flesh and plants tend to be much higher in potassium than sodium. Animals that eat a varied diet tend to be attracted to salt; the attraction of deer to a "salt lick" is an obvious example.

Our ancestors had access to a food supply naturally low in sodium. Sodium intake is essential for health, so natural selection would have led our ancestors to like the taste of salt. The salty foods to which they had access—seafood, some plants, the blood of animals—were generally desirable for other reasons as well, such as energy density or nutrient profile, thus lending additional reinforcement to any native preference for salty food.

In the modern world, our intake of sodium is generally far greater than that of potassium. While our ancestors are estimated to have consumed as much as ten times more potassium than sodium, we generally consume four or more times as much sodium as potassium!

Sodium enters the diet from diverse sources, including table salt (sodium chloride), baking soda (sodium bicarbonate), and flavor enhancers such as monosodium glutamate, to name a few. Salt curing of some products is still used for preservation. Thus, the modern food supply provides an abundance of sodium, which in conjunction with our native preference for it, contributes to excess intake of both sodium, and the foods in which it is particularly found.

Strategy

Sodium, or the salt in which it is found (sodium is a mineral that binds to another mineral, chloride, to make up salt), is both an intrinsic and acquired taste, meaning that we are predisposed to like salt from birth, but only actually come to like a high-salt intake after getting used to it.

Test Your Salt-Sensitivity

You can, in fact, demonstrate to yourself that you have adapted to a high-salt diet with a simple experiment—and this is a reasonable first step in devising a strategy to limit your salt intake. If you eat a commercial cereal regularly, such as *Cheerios* or *Corn Flakes*, you will probably not think of these as "salty" foods, even though the sodium content is considerable. If you convert from these cereals to their health-food counterparts (e.g., New Morning brand *Oatios*), which are low in sodium, for approximately two weeks, then retaste the commercial brand, you will indeed taste the salt. This will demonstrate how we condition ourselves not only to like salt, but to be relatively oblivious to its presence in our diets.

Counting Salt, Because Salt Counts

Whether or not you conduct the experiment, there are many things you can do to reduce your sodium intake. The first is to be aware of why some moderation in sodium intake is appropriate. There is evidence from international comparisons that more salt intake is associated with higher blood pressure; thus, if you have or are at risk for high blood pressure or vascular disease, sodium restriction makes good sense. Data from the DASH (*Dietary Approaches to Stop Hypertension*) study further indicate that sodium restriction, to about 1,200 mg per day, can significantly lower blood pressure, particularly when combined with a prudent overall dietary pattern based on grains, fruits, vegetables, and nonfat dairy. In addition, high-salt intake is associated with increased risk of osteoporosis, or thinning of the bones. And finally, salt can stimulate the satiety center for its taste in the brain, contributing to excess calorie intake.

The Saltshaker Fallacy

You must read food labels to moderate sodium intake because most sodium in the diet is in processed foods. The salt you add with a shaker contributes much less sodium to the average diet than the salt added in processing. In fact, there may be advantages to shaking salt on to your food. Salt added to food just prior to eating may be more readily tasted than salt added during preparation. In other words, a little salt added at the last minute may go a long way, while a lot added earlier may go less far.

Look for sodium in various forms on the ingredient label, and total sodium content on the nutrition label. As a reference, consider that if you eat 2,000 calories per day, and want to keep your sodium intake below the recommended maximum of 2.4 g per day, you should eat foods with less than 1.2 mg of sodium (Na) per calorie (120 mg for every 100 calories). If you are trying to reduce your sodium intake to the level achieved in the DASH trial, you need to eat foods with 60 mg of sodium per 100 kcal. If you eat too many processed foods with more than 1.2 mg of sodium per calorie, there is no way to keep your overall salt intake down to recommended levels.

Limiting Salt Intake, Naturally

While reading labels will help you know where sodium resides in your diet, it need not be a life's work! Natural, unprocessed foods, such as most vegetables, fruits, dried fruit, and whole grains are low in sodium. The more your diet is based on these foods, the lower your intake of sodium will be.

Some foods are very high in sodium, and really must be eaten in moderation to avoid sodium excess. Many of these foods—fast food, deli meats, cheese—are generally high in fat and calories as well, so again, efforts to moderate sodium intake will actually reinforce efforts to improve your overall dietary pattern. Some high-sodium foods, such as canned tuna, packaged soup, olives, and pickles, may be otherwise good for you. These foods are fine if part of a low-sodium diet, but can contribute to excessive sodium intake otherwise.

Less Salt, Same Satisfaction

Low-salt chips, soups, crackers, breads, cereals, dressings, spreads, and sauces are all readily available. These are an important part of efforts to reduce salt intake. Acclimate to salt-reduced foods slowly, knowing that as your intake goes down, so will your affinity for salt. Less salt intake generally leads to less salt preference, which makes further reductions, and/or maintaining the reductions already achieved, easier and easier with time.

Salt in Unsuspected Places

Most cakes, cookies, and other sweet baked goods contain considerable amounts of salt. The idea of a salty cookie may not be appealing, but this is indeed what most of us eat! Here, too, a trial of low-salt alternatives may taste a little bland at first, but if you stick it out for two weeks, then switch back, you will notice the salt in the products you ate before. In our experience, most people, once sensitized to taste the salt in baked goods, don't like it, and come to prefer the lower-salt alternatives.

Taking Advantage of Your Taste Buds

Other flavor enhancers can be used to mimic the taste of salt, without adding sodium to your diet. Citrus juices, particularly lemon and lime, partially mimic the taste and feel of salt on the tongue. Vinegar does as well. Some herbs, such as thyme, fennel, garlic, and rosemary, compensate admirably for reduced salt in many dishes (see Section IV for more detailed recommendations).

Obstacle/Opportunity 10
Pleasure/Gratification Induced by Food

Food is, and should be, a reliable source of pleasure. However, the pleasure from eating tends to act as positive reinforcement, encouraging more eating to generate more pleasure. This is perfectly normal— but can obviously lead us into some trouble as we try to control our waistlines!

There is a science devoted to the study of pleasure, called hedonics. The hedonics of food suggests that variation in pleasure responses to food may play a role in specific dietary choices. Some studies suggest that individuals susceptible to obesity, for example, may have heightened pleasure responses to dietary fat, leading to higher intake of calorie-dense foods.

The pleasure provided by food is complex. Chewing and eating can relieve tension. The taste of food stimulates pleasure, as does a feeling of fullness. The texture and consistency of food may also evoke pleasurable feelings. Certain foods, such as chocolate, tend to elicit very strong pleasure responses, at least in some people, for reasons not altogether understood. Beyond all of this, there are neurochemical responses to some foods and nutrients in the pleasure centers of our brains. These reactions, which are entirely beyond our control, can enhance the pleasure response to some foods in a very powerful way.

In addition to the pleasure responses to food that are built into our brains and our metabolism, there are pleasure responses built into our culture. Socially, food serves as an important focal point of gatherings and celebrations, and is thus linked to our memories of special events. This naturally associates food with good times, and with comfort during bad times. Culturally, food has long been a medium of art, as the term "culinary arts" suggests, adding the beauty of presentation to the pleasures of eating.

The Then/Now Conflict

For anyone subject to famine, eating is the difference between security and survival, and the threat of starvation. Naturally, then, eating has been a pleasurable activity throughout all of human history. In addition to pleasure obtained from filling an empty belly, our ancestors likely developed stronger pleasure responses to the particular foods and flavors that best supported their survival. The persistence of these Stone Age pleasure impulses in conjunction with modern ease of access makes the food "pleasure factor" a substantial barrier to healthful eating.

Strategy

In general, pleasure is good only up to a point. Any type of "over" indulgence is by very definition excessive, undesirable, and potentially harmful. Examples of our willingness to limit pleasure abound. Our society imposes constraints on the speed at which we drive, the ways we can behave in public, the use of alcohol, sexual activity, tobacco use, and many other potentially "pleasurable" activities. Illicit drugs such as cocaine reportedly evoke a strong sense of pleasure, yet most of us do not use such substances, and those that do wind up wishing they hadn't. The undisciplined pursuit of pleasure often leads to harm.

In this context, nutrition poses a unique challenge. Our society values abundance, and the practice of plate-cleaning. A feast or buffet is a delight to the eye and palate. We, quite naturally, find it difficult to think of the pleasure gained from eating, a life-sustaining activity, in the same light as, for example, drug use.

Too Much of a Good Thing

But, in fact, the strategy to manage the pleasure of food begins with just that kind of thinking. Too much pleasure leads to harm, and this is as true of food as it is of any other source.

Recall that in our society obesity is epidemic and worsening all the time, as is diabetes. Some four hundred thousand premature deaths each year relate directly or indirectly to obesity and the adverse effects of dietary excess. In this context, the long-term cost to health and well-being of food is often unacceptably high.

Accounting for Pleasure

Exactly how much pleasure from food is the "right" amount is something only you can decide. Keep in mind that food can cause both pleasure, and, in a sense, pain. If you eat food that tastes very good, you will enjoy it as you eat. But if your weight goes up to levels that make you unhappy, you will experience the pain of regret, and dissatisfaction.

Conversely, if you work hard to control your weight and diet, you may get pleasure from your appearance, or your health, but you may also feel sorry for yourself each time you forego eating a favorite food. There is a balance to be struck here. The immediate gratification of pleasurable foods should be adjusted relative to the long-term pleasure of maintaining a desirable weight, and good health. When you have that balance worked out for yourself, you have identified your own personal dietary pleasure *point of preference*. This is where you want to stay.

The Pleasure Trade-off. Pleasure is derived from eating favorite foods. However, as intake of these foods rises, weight may be gained and health compromised, reducing the pleasure from good health and weight control. The "point of preference" represents maximal pleasure when pleasure from eating, and from achieving good health and weight control are combined.

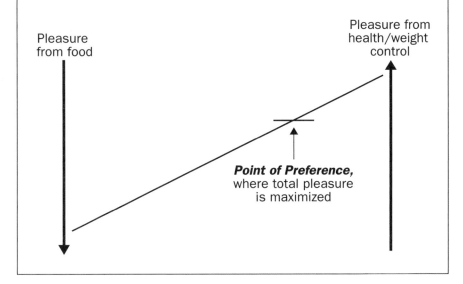

Pleasure from food

Pleasure from health/weight control

Point of Preference, where total pleasure is maximized

Protect Your Point of Preference

There are a variety of strategies to help you stay at your point of preference. First, as you are adjusting your diet to a more healthful pattern, consider the times in your day or week when eating your most pleasurable foods is most important to you. For example, you may tend to go out on weekends, or crave sweets after dinner. Begin by protecting these occasions as the time you will indulge yourself in highly pleasurable foods, such as chocolate, or cheese, or whatever your favorites happen to be (if your favorite food happens to be spinach, indulge any time you want!).

Protecting times and occasions for intensely pleasurable eating can help prevent you from feeling sorry for yourself as you make efforts to reach your point of preference. After all, you are not eliminating pleasure, you are maximizing it. Keep this in mind if ever you see someone eating some tempting food that you are resisting. Yes, the person eating that muffin, chocolate bar, slice of cake, or pizza may be experiencing pleasure at the moment—but they may wind up with the regret and discontent you would have afterward. If you are at or near your point of preference, and they are not, you are getting more total pleasure, not less, than they are.

Once the protected times are established, you must work to avoid being led into overindulgence at other times. One strategy for doing this is to rely on your food choices, rather than those of others. As discussed elsewhere, pack an insulated bag with healthful meals or snacks that you take with you every day. If and when you get hungry, eat something you prepared.

To avoid the temptation of other food exposures, decide in advance that they are simply off limits. If each time you pass a bakery counter or chocolate bar, or a coworker or friend says "try this," or you ask yourself "should I or shouldn't I?" sooner or later you will, whether you should or not! It is quite natural to eat the things we like when they are available, and unnatural to resist them. So no one is really strong enough to resist these temptations without a plan.

Plan Ahead; No Ropes Required

As noted earlier, Odysseus had himself lashed to the mast of his ship to resist the Sirens' call. Fortunately, you needn't lash yourself to anything other than your commitments! Decide in advance what foods are and are not acceptable at different times in your day or week, and lash yourself to these decisions. When a tempting food comes along, stick with the decision you've already made. If you need reinforcement in adhering to these types of commitments, consider sharing the commitments with a friend or confidante, who can then help to keep you on track.

Invest in Your Health

When you invest money, you are giving up the things that money could be spent on right away (i.e., giving up pleasure). But, protecting that money for the future means you can buy a house, or retire, or put your kids through college, and avoid the great displeasure of not being able

---

— Sad Sandy... —

Sandy, fifty-eight, had "dieted" many times, but always went off the diet, and gained back any weight she lost. For the most part, her weight gain was the result of feeling sorry for herself—watching other people eat foods that she was trying to give up. So she did give up— not the foods, but her efforts to control her weight.

But Sandy was, in a word, sad. Asked why, she said, "Isn't it obvious? Because I'm too fat!"

We gently helped Sandy to link this "sadness" to its source—the foods that were supposedly the source of pleasure she had been unwilling to give up! She "got it," and we worked toward a more suitable point of preference. The result—a lot more pleasure, a lot less sadness, and quite a few less pounds!

---

to do those things. Over the long-term, good investments result in gain, not loss, even though immediate pleasure is given up.

The same is true as you improve your eating habits. As a long-term strategy, the practice will actually reduce displeasure far more than pleasure, and move you toward your point of preference. The pleasure obtained from a healthful dietary pattern, leading to better health and weight control, will likely far outweigh the pleasure from eating whatever feels good. Thus, you gain the advantages of a healthful diet, while increasing, not decreasing, your net pleasure.

It isn't long before a dietary pattern that helps you maintain your point of preference is the way you are used to eating. At this point, there is no Siren song, or if there is, you no longer hear it. There is then no longer any need to lash yourself to your commitments. Rather, you can simply and safely sail past the hazard of intense dietary pleasures on the winds of your new *way to eat*.

Obstacle/Opportunity 11: Sensory Specific Satiety

Satiety, the sense of being full, is controlled by centers in a part of the brain called the hypothalamus. These centers are responsive to categories of taste (sweet, sour, salty, bitter). When satiety is reached in one taste category, appetite remains for the others; this is "sensory specific satiety."

You've experienced this whenever you felt full at the end of a large meal, but still had room for dessert! This trait is especially strong for sweet, the satiety threshold for which is higher than other tastes.

The Then/Now Conflict

Human health requires variety in the diet. We need protein, carbohydrate, and fat, along with vitamins, minerals, trace elements, and so on. To get all of these nutrients, we need to eat a range of foods. For us, this is as easy as a trip to a supermarket or cafeteria. For our ancestors, it was tough.

The tendency to feel full of one type of food or taste while still feeling hungry for others is thought to have protected our ancestors from nutrient deficiencies. Sensory specific satiety motivated them to have variety in their diets, even if it meant extra work.

Imagine, for example, if a herd of antelope took up residence in a valley next to our ancestral clan's cave. Easy hunting, to be sure, and very pleasant at first. Bur after a while, fore-mother, fore-father, and fore-kids probably said something a lot like, "What, antelope *again*??!!" Apparently, they got, quite literally, "fed up" with any one type of food, and were compelled by the satiety centers in their hypothalami (the controlling brain region), to seek variety. An essential tendency, because no one food provides all of the nutrients required by our metabolism.

Satiety thresholds are higher for sweets than for other flavors, and this is probably why dessert is taken at the end of the meal in almost all cultures. A craving for sweet may have been beneficial to our ancestors, because fruits and wild honey afforded a quick, convenient source of readily usable calories.

The modern food supply responds to our natural desire for dietary variety with both an astonishing variety of foods, and additional variety built into the ingredients of individual foods. As a result, we are stimulated to eat more, with food remaining appetizing for longer than it would if available in lesser variety. In this way, another prehistoric survival trait is turned against our efforts at healthful eating and moderation.

I Couldn't Eat Another Bite; What's for Dessert?

In discussing sensory-specific satiety, I am always inclined to mention the Katz family Thanksgiving. I will spare you the details, but suffice to say there is more food than three times as many guests could possibly eat, and all of it delicious. For me, to eat until I can eat no more, and then keep eating anyway, is simply a part of the tradition.

Yet even when the stuffing and potatoes I love become unappealing because I am just too stuffed myself, the dessert table still manages to appeal. In other words, "I couldn't eat another bite!" is followed, more or less immediately, by "What's for dessert?" That's the power of sensory specific satiety, not to mention Mom's cooking!

Strategy

Just knowing that you are influenced by sensory specific satiety is the first step toward dealing with it effectively. Being alerted to largely unperceived flavor enhancers added to commercial foods, such as salt in breakfast cereals, can help you limit their impact on your diet. You are already less susceptible to manipulation! But you must take some specific steps around this obstacle to dietary health.

One Food at a Time

Snacks should generally be comprised of one food, or a few closely related foods. On any given day, stick to a limited variety of snack foods from appropriate food categories (e.g., fresh fruit, fresh vegetables, whole-grain products, dried fruit, nonfat dairy, etc.).

Meals should be balanced, but not extravagant. While trying to control weight and energy intake, avoid buffets! Buffets interact with sensory specific satiety in a way that makes portion control nearly impossible for virtually everyone. In general, eat more "simple" foods in their natural state, and fewer processed (packaged) foods. The more ingredients processing adds to a food, the more likely it is to stimulate multiple satiety centers in the hypothalamus, rather than one, and the more you are likely to eat!

Variety Over Time, but Not Every Time

The influence of sensory specific satiety is at work over the course of a day, a week, or a year, but also during a single snack or meal. Satiety can be controlled in part by front-loading meals with filling, energy-dilute foods. Salad is a good example; the fiber content of vegetables tends to make them filling. This will often serve to blunt appetite for other components of the meal that tend to be more energy dense. Meals should be composed of several dishes (or even just one) with a somewhat common "taste" theme. The occasional feast of many diverse courses is a treat, but should not be routine if you have any interest in restraint.

There are various benefits of snacking provided that snacks are chosen from a relatively short list of foods (i.e., fresh fruit, dried fruit, fresh vegetables, whole-grain products, nonfat dairy). If you make excessive variety available to yourself, you may continue to enjoy eating longer than if you limit that variety.

Get Your Just Desserts

The satiety threshold for sweet is higher than for other flavors, so you will generally continue to find sweets appealing when all else ceases to be. To contend with this, make decisions about dessert before an array of choices tempts you.

If dealing with several options, choose one rather than more than one. Consider that an inclination for sweet can be satisfied as readily with nonfat sorbet as with high-fat ice cream; choose the lowest calorie, most nutritious option that will satisfy you. Establishing an overall dietary pattern that dictates when sweets will be part of a meal, and when not, is prudent. The rationale here in controlling behavioral responses is similar to the time-honored advice not to shop for food when hungry. An inability to resist dietary temptation is the norm, not the exception. Avoid temptation!

One (Per) Enchanted Evening

Sensory specific satiety has a particular interaction with evening snacking, and cravings. In efforts to control your calorie intake, you may attempt to avoid certain types of food, for example sweets, in the evening. Note that an appetite for a late evening snack may be produced

Don't Throw the Baby Out with the Bathwater...

One of the key strategies for dealing successfully with sensory specific satiety is to limit variety in your eating. However, eating a variety of foods—especially of natural foods—is important for balanced nutrition, and for getting all of the essential nutrients.

Limit the foods in any single meal or snack as a means of controlling appetite. But vary the grains, fruits, vegetables, seeds, beans, nuts, dairy products, and meats you eat over time to get a wide array of nutrients in your diet.

or accentuated by a brisk insulin release in response to a large evening meal. This is an additional reason among those already discussed to snack in the afternoon and moderate the size of dinner.

Some tendency for snacking in the evening is common, however, even if the evening meal is moderate. If you tend to like a late-evening snack, you should make particular plans to contend with sensory specific satiety.

Set a cut-off time, typically at least two hours before sleep, after which you don't eat. In addition to this, make certain that you restrict to just one snack food each evening. The greatest risk of overindulgence comes from eating one type of food, moving on to another, and so on. Plan the choices in advance as much as possible. You can rotate choices by day of the week, for example, if you like an orderly schedule.

On the other hand, if you have an occasional strong craving, you are generally well advised to give in to it directly. The common experience with cravings is that they are persistent as you try to address them with your choices rather than theirs, and then they still win in the end. Rather than eating an assortment of foods and ending with the craved food, go to it directly if it's available, and have nothing else.

Surfing the Urge
If you find that you are having urges, or cravings for food that you would rather resist than give in to, there is a strategy that addiction specialists

use that can help. It's called "urge surfing." The basic concept is that any craving builds, and then dissipates, like a wave. Just as surfers "catch" a wave to ride its power rather than be tossed around by it, you can ride through cravings for foods you are trying to limit. Picture a wave in your mind, and let it build as the craving builds, knowing that it will peak. As you near the peak intensity of the craving, comfort yourself by knowing that the only thing that can happen next is for the craving to start to fade; no craving lasts forever! Picture the wave curling, then falling on the sand; it's over. Way to go, "Dude"! You've surfed the urge! Once you know how to do this, and have done it successfully, cravings lose their power to intimidate you, or toss you around.

Gain Insight into Food Industry Practices

The challenge of sensory specific satiety is compounded by the practices of the modern food industry, which knows a good deal about our tastes, traits, and tendencies. Examples of industry exploitation of this particular trait abound. Breakfast cereals, not generally eaten as "salty" food, often contain nearly as much sodium per serving as potato or corn chips. The taste of the salt is masked by the sugar content, but likely stimulates the taste center in the hypothalamus just the same. As discussed above, a preference for salt-laden cereal is learned, and can be unlearned.

Other baked goods have added salt. What we tend to think of as salty foods, such as ketchup, have added sugar. And many processed foods have long ingredient lists that introduce a wide range of flavor influences, many of them so subtle we are not aware of them, while our satiety centers doubtless are.

To contend with this, you will once again be well served by reading food labels. Many of the same selections that help you limit your intake of dietary fat or salt will help you limit the unnecessary variety of ingredients introduced into your diet. Once you have familiarized yourself with the products that avoid unnecessary additions of sugar, salt, or chemical flavor modifiers, the hard part is over. You need no longer read food labels, but rather just continue to use the products you have selected (see Section IV for a head start). Only the transition period to an improved dietary pattern is highly effort dependent; maintenance is generally fairly easy.

Beware the Tangled Web of Obstacles

Many of the challenges to eating well interact with one another, creating a virtual "obstacle course," or a web of challenges. For example, the lure of dietary fat contributes to the lure of excessive dietary variety, and vice versa. Sweet is pleasurable, and many foods are both sweet and fatty, with the sweet encouraging even greater fat intake than would otherwise occur.

But the good news is that the strategies useful for confronting any single challenge to eating well also interact with multiple obstacles, almost invariably confronting several, many, or even all at once, converting them into opportunities for progress along the *way to eat*. The strategies adopted for overcoming each of the many obstacles to nutritional health come together to confront them all, the whole approach being greater than the sum of its individual parts.

Obstacle/Opportunity 12
Variations in Resting (Basal) Metabolism

Basal metabolism, known by various other terms including resting energy expenditure (REE), is the energy cost of living. As you read this, your heart is pumping, blood is flowing. Your lungs are working like bellows. Your liver is detoxifying the blood, your kidneys are filtering it. And so on. Each of these functions comes with an energy cost. Every cell in the body is consuming energy constantly.

The food we eat provides energy to support this "basal" activity, as well as the work of our muscles. Additionally, some energy is wasted in the generation of heat; no machine is perfectly efficient in its use of energy, and the human body is no exception. The loss of energy as heat tends to occur in particular following meals and is referred to as *postprandial thermogenesis*, or the "thermogenesis of food."

In general, the work of muscles and postprandial thermogenesis each contributes roughly 15 percent to total daily energy expenditure. The contribution of physical activity to energy use, of course, varies with the level of physical activity. But for most of us, a full 70 percent of energy ingested is used in support of basal metabolism.

The energy required to maintain basal metabolism varies with body size, and in particular, muscle mass, just as it requires the burning of more fuel to maintain constant temperature in a large building than in a small one. What tends to be frustrating is that even among people of more or less identical size and build, basal metabolism varies.

The result of this variation is a line often heard when one provides dietary counseling: "I eat nothing and still gain weight." Or: "I eat less than so-and-so, and they stay thin, while I gain weight." These impressions are, in general, at least partially true.

The reasons metabolic rate varies among individuals are not fully worked out, but a genetic basis is clear. In some ethnic groups, adaptation to a particular diet and environment has resulted in extreme metabolic efficiency, or a low basal metabolism. In conjunction with a high-calorie food supply and limited physical activity, a low basal metabolism becomes an important barrier to weight control.

The Then/Now Conflict

For our ancestors, there was a survival advantage in being "fuel-efficient," a particularly important aspect of which is the capacity to maintain the activity of the body's billions of cells at a minimal energy cost. Therefore, a low resting energy expenditure, or basal metabolic rate, was doubtless favored by the forces of natural selection.

Not all of our ancestors would have exactly the same basal metabolic rate, any more than they would all be identical in any other way. What would tend to happen, though, is that the entire species would be *relatively* fuel efficient. Those peoples living in, and adapting to, places where food was in especially short supply might tend to be at the extreme end of the metabolic efficiency scale. Those peoples adapting to more plentiful surroundings would perhaps tend to be somewhat less efficient, falling at the other end of the spectrum.

In the modern world, when fuel (food) is plentiful, a low rate of basal metabolism results in susceptibility to weight gain, and the many consequences of being overweight and suffering from obesity.

Strategy

One of the first challenges encountered when contending with a low basal metabolism is the need for legitimacy. A great many of my patients have felt compelled to "convince" me that their metabolic rate was low. I believe them! I think they may have been trying to convince

— Laura's Lament: —

"I only need to *smell* food to gain weight!"

themselves, and perhaps you are, too. So, know that it is true. Basal metabolism does vary, and many people subject to weight gain have a relatively low basal metabolic rate (BMR).

Another challenging component of the influence of BMR on weight regulation is the sense of injustice. If you eat less, or exercise more, than someone else who stays thin while you don't—it is likely to tick you off!

Don't feel persecuted. There is no reason why weight regulation should be "fair." If you are metabolically efficient, you are likely the descendant of a group of people for whom metabolic efficiency was essential. If they had not been fuel efficient, they would not have survived, and you wouldn't be here! So, when next feeling sorry for yourself about your metabolism, consider that the alternative might be never having been born.

People Are Different
Accept that people vary in many ways. In a room at some given temperature, some people will feel comfortable, others too cold, others too warm. We vary in our emotional responses, our sensitivity, and our insight. Why shouldn't we vary in our BMR?

So, accept that your BMR is what it is, and get on with business. If you have a low BMR, you can compensate in a variety of ways. The first, and most basic, is to reduce your energy intake. Like a fuel-efficient car, you will go farther than most on less fuel, so take in less fuel. Restrict your intake of dietary fat because fat is energy dense. Control your portion sizes. Snack on appropriate foods to control your appetite and help you keep total energy intake moderate.

Mind Your Own Basal Metabolic Business
Appreciate that weight control is always a product of achieving balance between energy taken in, and energy used up. If your energy

expenditure is low due to a low BMR, your intake must be comparably low, or you *will* gain weight. Don't compare your level of food intake to anyone else's as a basis for deciding what's appropriate. Your BMR is unique to you, so the level of fuel intake your body needs for weight maintenance is also unique to you. It will likely be more than is needed by some, less than is needed by some others. What's right for you is what's right for you.

In addition to reducing your energy intake, you can, of course, increase your energy expenditure. The more physically active you are, the more fuel you burn. Exercise alone, however, is often not sufficient to produce weight loss, even though it is *very important* for both weight maintenance, and overall health. Basal metabolism consumes approximately 1–1.5 kcal per minute in an adult of average size. Moderate walking can triple or even quadruple this energy consumption, while very vigorous activity, such as running or swimming freestyle, can increase it by a factor of thirty or more.

Consider what happens if you walk at a moderately fast pace for an hour a day in an effort to control your weight. During that hour, your BMR would burn 1.5 kcal per minute, or 90 kcal, if you weren't walking. The walking increases your energy consumption by a factor of 4, so during that same hour, you burn about 6 kcal/minute, or 360 kcal. The net "gain" in calories burned is 360–90, or 270 kcal. Over the course of a week, if you kept all of your other activities and your diet constant, this level of activity would result in the loss of roughly 1/2–1/3 pound!

So, you could commit to walking an hour a day, which is quite a lot of walking, and still lose only 1/3 of a pound per week. Further, BMR varies with body mass. As you lose weight, your BMR goes down! If your BMR drops from 1.5 kcal per minute to, for example, 1 kcal per minute, that same hour of walking will only burn 240 kcal, and the net gain in calories burned will only be 180 kcal. And so on.

But don't despair! This dose of reality is not meant to be bad news. If you have unrealistic expectations about the results of exercise, or about your efforts to control weight, you are likely to become discouraged and give up. Be realistic about weight control: it's difficult, and BMR is an important consideration.

Less In, More Out

While physical activity alone, unless at a very high level, is unlikely to compensate for low BMR in your efforts to control your weight, in combination with other strategies it can be very effective. As noted above, work to reduce the energy density of your diet, and your portion sizes. Simply by taking sugar and cream (e.g., Half & Half) out of several cups of coffee a day, you could save as many calories as spent in walking for an hour. Do both, and you have doubled the benefits. Take fat and calories out of your diet in several other places, and you profit further.

Your Metabolism in Motion

If you are physically active enough to increase your muscle tone and muscle mass somewhat, you will actually increase your BMR, or if you are losing weight, at least maintain your BMR. Improve your muscle tone by working toward the recommended thirty minutes or more of moderate activity on most days (at least five times per week), and by combining aerobic activities with strength, or resistance activities, such as weight lifting, calisthenics, or isometrics. If in addition to any exercise you do, you also make an effort to be physically active during your daily routine by using stairs instead of the elevator, walking down the hall instead of using an intercom, parking in the farthest rather than closest space, etc., you will gain additional benefits. Make being "kinetic," or a person known for being always in motion, a goal and a source of pride.

Taking Fate into Your Own Hands

Little by little, these incremental changes in your lifestyle can and will compensate for a low BMR. But the successful strategy begins with a clear understanding of the obstacle. A low BMR is not a character flaw, nor a genetic defect. It is a natural by-product of a long prehistoric struggle with a limited food supply. Also, keep in mind that a low BMR is not something you can ever fully change. This is one of the reasons why short-term dieting makes no sense. Even if you lose weight, you will not have changed the underlying tendency to gain weight. Gradual adjustments to your diet and lifestyle that you can live with forever are the appropriate way of responding to, and managing, a BMR you will also be living with forever.

If an unusually low BMR is interfering with weight control, testing for a metabolic disorder, and/or use of medication, might be considered. Drugs for weight control, both prescription and nonprescription, are described briefly in Section IV. Their use is not recommended unless obesity represents a health threat not controllable by other means. If you are struggling with control of your weight in part due to a low BMR, you should certainly discuss it with your doctor or a dietitian. If medication is used, it should always be in addition to, and never instead of, prudent dietary and physical activity practices, both because medication is unlikely to work alone, and because no pill can offer the many benefits of a health-promoting lifestyle.

Obstacle/Opportunity 13
Variations in Body Type/Fat Deposition

While we are almost all subject to weight gain when food is abundantly available, and physical activity is optional, our susceptibilities are variable. Some people gain weight very easily, others somewhat less so. Some people can go for long periods without eating and feel no ill effects, others have symptoms after fasting for only short periods.

Another important variant is the distribution of body fat. Men are generally more susceptible than women to the accumulation of weight around the middle, referred to rather unglamorously as a "beer belly." In clinical circles, this pattern of weight gain is referred to as "central adiposity," the "android" pattern of obesity, or the "apple pattern."

Women are more susceptible than men to weight gain in the buttocks, thighs, and lower extremities. This pattern is referred to as the "gynoid" or "pear" pattern of obesity. Neither of these patterns is truly gender specific; some men are subject to the gynoid pattern, and some women to the android pattern.

There is much more to this story than meets the eye. Fat that tends to accumulate around the middle—the android pattern—is associated with a tendency to accumulate fat in and around vital organs. This fat is generally rich in a type of receptor, the beta-3 adrenergic receptor, that is a binding site for epinephrine and related "stimulant" hormones. These hormones interact with the fat tissue in a way that tends to raise blood pressure and increase cardiac risk. In fact, while obesity is a clearly established risk factor for cardiovascular disease, this is true only for abdominal, or central obesity. Fat distributed in the lower extremities is not associated with an increased risk of heart disease.

The difference between the android and gynoid patterns is often apparent upon casual inspection, but can also be measured with the "waist-to-hip ratio." When the measure around the waist is high relative to the measure around the hips, there is central obesity. When the hips are large relative to the waist, central obesity can generally be ruled out.

While the beta-3 adrenenergic receptor in centrally distributed fat contributes to cardiac risk, it does have a redeeming characteristic: it makes fat loss relatively easy. When calorie intake is restricted, centrally distributed fat is lost fairly readily. In contrast, lower extremity fat stores are relatively resistant to calorie restriction.

This, of course, tends to frustrate a lot of people, especially women, particularly those with gynoid obesity married to husbands with android obesity. When both "go on a diet" together, the man loses weight quickly, the woman does not. This is a natural and unavoidable by-product of physiologic differences you probably didn't know were at work.

The Then/Now Conflict

Not everything about human metabolism is readily explained by invoking the evolutionary biology model. In the case of body fat distribution, there is no ironclad evidence of an evolutionary role. However, there is a very plausible explanation for the tendency of women to gain fat in a way that is both safe, and resistant to calorie restriction.

All weight gain in the form of fat is a defense against dietary shortfalls. Fat is an energy reserve. The normal human condition that calls for the greatest energy reserve is pregnancy. Being able to store fat safely and efficiently, in a manner relatively resistant to rapid turnover, would very likely have been beneficial to women bearing children, and subject to famine throughout prehistory. While needing to store fat for their own survival, men would not need to create so stable and durable an energy reserve, and might well benefit from a depot of fat more readily available for use as fuel. This theory might well account for the well-established differences in weight gain and loss patterns observed in women and men.

In modern context, fat depots tend to persist. Fat stored in more stable reserves, typically in the lower extremities, is particularly hard to lose without extreme effort.

Strategy

Abdominal, or centrally distributed fat, is relatively easy to lose. It is also especially important to lose, as it so clearly contributes to insulin resistance and cardiovascular risk. If subject to this pattern of weight gain, efforts at weight control are especially important.

Be Realistic

For those—often, but by no means always, women—subject to lower extremity weight gain, an important first step is realistic expectations. Many women with this predisposition actually cannot achieve truly thin hips, buttocks, and thighs without being thinner than they care to be in the face and upper body. If you are in this category, you will probably need to reconcile yourself to carrying some lower extremity weight that you would prefer to lose. Far better to accept a few extra pounds, and understand that doing so is in no way a failure, than to make the loss of those pounds an unhappy, lifelong obsession.

You Win Some When You Lose Some

To lose some, or perhaps even all, excess lower extremity weight, a combination of exercise and restriction of calorie intake is generally necessary. Of course, restricting calorie, or "energy" intake is needed to achieve weight loss anywhere in the body. The loss of weight cannot really be directed to any one body part, and fat will first be burned from the depots that are most "metabolically accessible." This is the reason why some people can be thinner than desired in one body part, while still heavier than desired in another.

Here is where exercise comes in. By exercising a particular area of the body, muscle tone and mass are both increased. This tends to result in improvements in body contour and appearance, while to some extent helping to mobilize fat. Thus, while hopes for targeted, or localized weight loss tend to be unrealistic, using exercise in combination with appropriate dietary practices can help achieve some degree of body "sculpting." But don't forget that you are not made of clay; your body will have the final say. Combine your good efforts with realistic expectations, and a willingness to accept the things you can't change—and you'll not only be thinner and healthier, but also a lot more content!

The Proverbial Ounce of Prevention

For many, and perhaps for you, the option of weight gain prevention may have already come and gone. But whenever possible, applying this strategy is far preferable to the alternatives. A lifetime of healthful lifestyle practices can prevent excess fat deposition in the first place.

This option is, of course, most consistently relevant to children, so even as you read this for your own sake, consider sharing the messages with your children, your nieces, nephews, or grandchildren. Children benefit from eating well and being physically active, just as adults do. But by starting these practices early, children enjoy the additional potential benefit of avoiding undesired fat deposition in the first place. For some adults, this remains a viable option. Keeping fat off is generally easier, and more effective, than taking fat off, so the earlier one adopts a health-promoting lifestyle, the better.

Combining an understanding of the variations in body fat deposition with realistic expectations about weight control, and prudent applications of diet and exercise, can help you achieve satisfactory management of this challenging issue.

Obstacle/Opportunity 14
Variations in Taste Sensitivity

The taste of food, which in fact depends quite heavily on the sense of smell in addition to the sense of taste, influences what we like and don't like, what we do and don't eat. There is evidence that sensitivity to taste varies, and that some people are "super tasters." Sensitivity to taste may be linked to heightened pleasure from food, an increased susceptibility to excessive intake, and weight gain.

The Then/Now Conflict

Taste, along with smell and sight, was what our ancestors used to distinguish familiar from unfamiliar food, safe food from poison. Acuity in the sense of taste would naturally tend to vary just as visual acuity, auditory acuity, and other human traits do. An acute sense of taste might well have been advantageous to our ancestors in their efforts to select safe foods, and avoid toxins in plants. In modern context, an especially acute sense of taste may stimulate appetite, and contribute to overeating, or cause aversions.

Strategy

First, if you get intense pleasure or displeasure from the flavor of certain foods, consider that you might be a "super taster." Testing for this trait is possible in research settings, but isn't really necessary. If you think you might be a super taster, there's no harm in assuming you are.

Understand that this trait may tend to cause you to eat more calories than you need. Controlling this tendency is important for weight control and dietary health.

Control Your Exposures

Identify those foods that give you particularly intense pleasure, and limit your exposure to them. Base your diet mostly on nutrient-dense, energy-dilute foods, such as whole-grain products, vegetables, and fruit. Have these foods readily available, and snack on them liberally to keep your appetite in check. If necessary, make specific commitments, and engage in some social contracting to help control your intake of foods that tend to overpower your restraint.

Limit your intake of intensely pleasurable foods to settings and times chosen in advance. Sticking to such commitments will be most challenging at first, getting easier with time as changes in your dietary pattern become more established and familiar. Don't shop for food or attend social gatherings that might lead you into undesired "dietary temptation" when you are hungry; eat nutritious, calorie-dilute snacks in advance of these activities. Use your food diary to alert you to those times and places where you are most vulnerable to overeating.

To avoid a sense of deprivation, don't remove favorite foods from your diet altogether; simply control the context in which you consider it reasonable to indulge. Eating should be pleasurable, and the inclusion of intensely pleasurable foods in the diet is both reasonable and important. However, intense pleasure and restraint tend to be at odds with one another. Therefore, controlling the frequency, quantity, and context of dietary indulgences is necessary for good health.

Keep the Taste, Cut the Calories

One additional strategy that can help satisfy an acute sense of taste, while avoiding the harm that can come from doing so, is to use food substitutions in which the primary taste is preserved. If, for example, you love chocolate, switching to fat-reduced cakes or cookies, or from ice cream to sorbet, will still permit you access to the flavor of chocolate, while helping you avoid fat and calories.

Obstacle/Opportunity 15: Weight Loss Plateau

Frustration is an enemy to all good intentions, and frustration in weight control is nearly universal. Often, the most intense frustration and disappointment occur during an effort at weight loss when, after initial success, weight suddenly plateaus and won't budge. At this point, many people abandon their weight-control effort altogether.

These weight-loss plateaus are perfectly normal, and easily explained. Basal metabolism accounts for approximately 70 percent of all calories burned by the body, and is dependent on body mass. When weight loss occurs, body mass goes down; so, too, does basal metabolic rate (BMR).

Consider an example: you eat a 2,000 kcal diet, weigh 176 lbs (80kg) and would like to lose 20 lbs at a rate of 1 lb per week. For purposes of this example, consider as well that you have a BMR of 1.2 kcal per minute, and burn 150 kcal per day in physical activity, and another 100 or so as heat loss (postprandial thermogenesis). The BMR accounts for 1,728 kcal per day (1.2 X 60 X 24), and added up, total energy use in a twenty-four-hour period is 1,978 kcal, roughly equivalent to the 2,000 kcal intake. When calories taken in equal calories burned, weight remains stable.

To lose 1 lb a week requires that the number of calories in 1 lb of body fat be taken out of the diet each week. One pound of body fat is 454 grams of fat, each of which has 9 kcal, for a total of just over 4,000 kcal. Thus, the loss of 1 lb per week requires a calorie deficit of roughly 4,000 kcal per week, or between 500 and 600 kcal per day.

So, you begin this weight-loss effort by cutting your calorie intake by 25 percent, from 2,000 kcal per day, to 1,500 kcal per day. At first, all goes well, and you do indeed lose weight at a pound a week. But after about six weeks, you hit a plateau. This is because with the weight loss, your BMR has now fallen. Assume that it has declined from 1.2 kcal per minute, to 0.9 kcal per minute. The total daily energy cost of BMR is now 1,296 kcal. Add to this the 250 kcal used in heat loss and physical activity, and the total, 1,546 kcal, is very close to your new daily intake! This means you've hit a new equilibrium, and won't lose any more weight unless you decrease calories taken in, increase calories burned, or both.

The Then/Now Conflict

It makes sense that basal metabolism should fall when weight loss occurs. For one thing, it is inevitable, as BMR is a product of the activity of the body's cells; if the number or size of those cells declines, so does the total level of cellular activity. For another, it is an appropriate response in evolutionary context. Weight loss for our ancestors was almost certainly never the result of intent, but rather the undesired result of having too little to eat. Under those circumstances, weight loss might indicate a threat of starvation. A logical defense against starvation is a reduction in the body's energy requirements. The less energy expended daily, the longer one could survive with limited, or no, food intake.

Of course, our physiology is not designed to distinguish between the threat of starvation and intentional weight loss; the metabolic reaction to both is the same. In modern context, this physiologic response makes the already difficult challenge of weight control even more difficult and frustrating.

Strategy

Be realistic about weight loss. Most interventions promising rapid weight loss are not sustainable, and thus tend to confer little long-term benefit. If you are intent on weight loss, a rate of one to at most two pounds per week is generally appropriate.

Ed's Explanation...

Ed, thirty-five, was pretty committed to weight loss, and was in fact, doing all the right things. Except one: he was focused on weight, rather than health. He was eating better, even being more active, and losing weight—for a while. But when he hit a weight-loss plateau, he felt like he was failing. Even though he still had all the benefits of a more healthful lifestyle, Ed looked only at the scale for evidence of success.

Worse, still, he felt as if he needed to explain why he wasn't losing weight. "Really, doc, I'm still eating better! I am..."

Of course, I believed him—he just didn't believe himself! We talked about plateaus, and about focusing on eating well and being active more than on weight. In Ed's case, that was the needed formula. He relaxed, and settled into his new and healthy lifestyle. The more he got used to the new *way*, the better he did with it. As a result, he even got beyond the weight-loss plateau. Ed now worries less about his weight and focuses on his lifestyle. But as a fringe benefit of doing so, he actually weighs just about what he wants to!

The Weight-loss Terrain

Anticipate that you will hit plateaus in your weight-loss effort. Don't be frustrated by them; they are inevitable. When you hit a plateau, decide whether or not further weight loss is worth additional effort. If not, concentrate on weight maintenance or health rather than weight. Whatever your weight, eating well and being physically active are good for you! If you are committed to more weight loss, you will need to make further adjustments in your energy balance to succeed. This can be done by further reducing calorie intake, increasing energy expenditure in the form of physical activity, or both.

To Keep Going, Get Going

Increasing physical activity is a particularly useful strategy in sustaining weight loss and moving below a plateau, because exercise both uses calories and builds muscle. The more muscle you have, the higher your basal metabolic rate. If you do increase your muscle mass slightly as you lose body fat, it can compensate for the decline in BMR induced by weight loss, and keep you in negative energy balance. Negative energy balance is when you are burning more calories than you are taking in, and is necessary for weight loss to occur.

There is limited, preliminary evidence that shifting some calories from carbohydrate or fat to protein may help preserve BMR during weight loss. Even if this is so, the effect is apparently modest. An increase in protein intake up to 20 percent or so of calories is a reasonable strategy to maintain weight loss; at higher levels of protein intake, the risks are likely to outweigh any benefits.

By improving your eating habits, and increasing your physical activity level, you will almost certainly lose weight. If and when you hit a weight-loss plateau, you don't lose the benefits of your healthier lifestyle, or of the weight you've already lost. Maybe you can keep going, or maybe you'll just maintain your new, lower weight. Either way, recognize that a healthier lifestyle in and of itself is a great success.

Step 4:

Dismiss Misinformation, Fend off Folklore

FOOD HAS ALWAYS been at the very heart of social activity. Food, eating, and health are talked about on radio and television, in magazines and newspapers, on the Internet, and at the water cooler. Whenever we gather with friends or family, a focal point, if not *the* focal point, is food.

The importance of food to human society has resulted in a great deal of folklore about ways we should, or should not, eat. The competing and diverse interests of food consumers, food producers, weight-loss programs, diet authors, and the media have resulted in the generation of a great many misleading messages. This mass of misinformation is a potent challenge to eating well.

The most powerful way to dismiss misinformation is to have good information in its place. You need to know what constitutes a health-promoting diet. You need to know the composition of your diet, and be able to assess the composition of various foods within any given category. You need to know when someone is trying to sell you the proverbial "bill of goods." You also need to know that misinformation abounds, and be alert to its threat. Just knowing this vulnerability goes a long way toward eliminating it.

This Step teaches you to blend skills acquired in some of the earlier steps into strategies that will help you steer a safe course through a sea of misinformation, folklore, and social influences, including:

1) *Challenges in Satisfying Other Family Members'*
   Food Preferences

2) *Children's Dietary Patterns and Preferences*

3) *Conflicting Messages by "Experts"*

4) *Costs, or Perceptions Regarding Costs, of Nutritious Foods*

5) *Folklore: Danger of "Skipping" Breakfast*

6) *Folklore: Hazards of Snacking*

7) *Food Categorization or Generalization*

8) *Food Inattentiveness*

9) *Inability to Interpret Food Labels*

10) *Sabotage, Well-meaning & Otherwise*

11) *Social "Normalization" of Being Overweight*

12) *Starting Tomorrow: The Scarlett O'Hara Syndrome*

13) *The Burden of Nutritional "Virtue"*

14) *Time Constraints That Limit Physical Activity*

15) *Use of Food as Basis for Social Gatherings*

Obstacle/Opportunity 1: Challenges in Satisfying Other Family Members' Food Preferences

We are social creatures, and little we do is more social than eating. For many modern families, dinner remains the one time in the day when people gather. Most of our special events, holidays, and celebrations are built largely around food. As a result, the conflicting food preferences of our social group can make choosing and sticking with an improved dietary pattern even more challenging than it already is. This is particularly so if the conflicts occur within the "nuclear family," those people living with us, with whom we share meals every day.

To adopt a healthful diet for yourself, and not need a different diet/meal plan for every member of the family, requires that the approach to diet and health be generalizable to the rest of your family.

The Then/Now Conflict

Prehistoric, hunter-gatherer families probably ate together as we do. But what they ate was less a matter of choice than of necessity. Often, only just enough food was available. Under those circumstances, it was easy, in fact unavoidable, for family groups to eat a common diet.

In the modern world, we have all been exposed to a vast array of dietary options. If you do not engage your family in a healthful way of eating, you are left with unpleasant choices: abandon your efforts, or eat differently from the rest of your family. The latter option is both unpleasant and inconvenient, and the former even worse!

Strategy

We assume as we offer these strategies that your family is willing to be supportive of you, as well as their own goals for diet, weight, and health.

Family Power

Begin by enlisting the support of your family. Be very clear that you are working to improve your diet, weight, and health. In the case of your significant other, let them know that you will need their help and support. You can also identify the ways in which similar dietary modifications will be beneficial for them.

As for children, depending on their ages, you will need to use your own judgment about how to get them actively involved. Very small children will, of course, not understand your efforts at dietary change, but don't need to. Small children change their diets quite readily, and will just come along for the ride!

Children old enough to have strong opinions about their preferences require a different approach. Let them know what you are doing and why, and explain it in terms relevant to them. Most parents accept the need to discuss the risks of smoking, sex, alcohol, and drugs with their children, and all health experts encourage having these discussions. In a society where obesity and diabetes are epidemic in our children, isn't it time to add nutrition (and physical activity) to the list? Many more children are harmed, over their lifetime, by poor diets than by drugs. In our view, it is indeed time to have these discussions. Make sure they are balanced, though. The focus should be on health, not weight. Undue preoccupation with weight control is one of the factors associated with eating disorders, especially in girls.

Help your kids to understand that a healthful diet is as essential for them as it is for you. But then, back off just a bit. Let your family know that this won't be a sudden, radical overhaul of the family diet—that you are not about to become the nutrition police. Make a commitment to strategize together, and to support one another. Identify those dietary changes the family is most willing to make, and adopt those first.

Let everyone know that new, more healthful foods will require a one to two week transition period, but if after that they remain opposed, you will be prepared to compromise. Any changes you make toward a more healthful diet will benefit you and your family; you do not need to be dogmatic about every change you try.

Know Your Options

Become familiar with healthful alternatives to your family's favorite foods, such as baked rather than fried chips, fat-free dairy products, and fat-reduced desserts. Use these substitutions to help retain the types of foods your family prefers, while improving their overall eating habits. Use ingredient substitutions to do the same with dishes prepared at home.

Through a combination of candor, commitment, and compromise, you can make your new way of eating your family's new way of eating, to the benefit of all.

Obstacle/Opportunity 2
Children's Dietary Patterns and Preferences

Children are just as subject to the dietary preferences that compromise health as adults are, and they lack adult restraint and adult insight. Children also tend to be even more averse to new foods and flavors than adults. So, accommodating your kids can pose quite a challenge as you try to improve the way you eat.

Bad dietary habits established in childhood generally predict such habits throughout life, increasing the risk for diet-related health problems in adulthood. Good eating habits in childhood also tend to predict later behavior. Because of this, helping to achieve good eating habits in childhood is especially important.

The Then/Now Conflict

In the prehistoric world, and throughout most of history, children ate what their parents could provide, or they starved. In the modern world, all of our dietary preferences can be indulged. Because familiarity is a strong determinant of food preferences, once a high-fat, high-sugar, high-salt diet has been adopted, the familiarity of that dietary pattern reinforces its appeal. Kids tend to like sugar, salt, and fat to begin with, as we all do, and learn to like them even more because they eat them all the time.

Strategy

Recognize that while children may be less motivated to change their diets than adults, they actually adapt to change more readily. The younger children are, the more easily they tend to acclimate to new dietary patterns. So, there will never be a better time than today to begin improving the dietary practices of your kids.

Sometimes, You're the Boss…

If your children are too young to understand the rationale for trying to eat a healthful diet, they are young enough to have dietary changes imposed without much discussion. Use the strategies and skills imparted throughout this book to make your home a "safe" nutritional environment. In this environment, you can still provide all of the food types your children are likely to request, including cookies, snacks, and chips. Children wanting ice cream in a home that only stocks nonfat frozen yogurt, or sorbet, will not know the difference! (As a father of five children, I know this from personal experience.)

Of course, maintaining such practices will be easier than establishing them. Children, like adults, will tend to resist any dietary change. But they can acclimate. Stick with your plan, and your new foods, for two weeks, putting up with any protests during that time. You will likely notice by the end of that period that the fussing is over. For guidance on the many food substitutions worth considering, see Section IV.

…Sometimes, You're Not

If your children are old enough to understand the link between diet and health, discuss it with them. They may already have a weight problem, and if not, will certainly have friends who do. Children are generally no happier about being overweight than adults, and equally prone to stigma and ridicule by their peers, if not more so.

In fact, in an experiment conducted in kindergartens in the U.S., children were shown photos of other children with various characteristics: ethnic dress, glasses, a wheelchair, crutches, or obesity. Asked which of these kids they would least like to play with, 95 percent of the children polled select the obese child. Clearly, we are imparting a very unfortunate prejudice to our children. But equally clear, no kid wants to be obese if they can help it. And they can.

In the same nonjudgmental way that you would like your own dietary habits addressed, help your children to understand that the way they eat will influence their health. Identify healthful eating as a family priority, something to work toward, and take pride in. Tell them you need their help, and will provide them yours. Make eating well a family commitment.

And We Helped!

One good way of getting young kids interested in eating well is to involve them in food preparation. Let them help you prepare the dishes you particularly want to introduce into their diets. Because they feel responsible for these dishes, they will be more likely to taste them, and to try to like them.

Look Out for…You

As you work to develop family consensus in favor of eating well, pay particular attention to the ways you might be sabotaging your own efforts! Consider that some of the basis for your own struggle with dietary health comes from your own experience as a child.

In both animals and humans, dietary patterns learned even before birth, during breast-feeding, and in childhood tend to track into adulthood. Many of the dietary habits that make it so hard for you to control your weight were probably taught to you when you were a child. Your mother, for example, probably urged you to clean your plate. Why? One generation has passed along to the next—from the Paleolithic era to the Dark Ages right up to the Depression and beyond— the fear of not having enough food, and parents can't seem to get used to the idea that in the modern era of epidemic obesity, the danger is eating too much rather than too little.

If you traditionally encourage plate-cleaning, it's time to stop. That is a practice held over from eons of dietary deprivation. When we all have too much to eat, there is no good reason for eating all we have! Encourage your children to eat until full. Put less on their plates, rather than asking them to eat more.

Recognize that children may eat erratically, but do not starve themselves. There is good evidence that nutrient and energy needs are met by children over a span of several days, even if not met every day. Allow your children to develop a comfortable relationship with food. To the extent that you can, let them eat when they are hungry, and as much as they want. Be sure to give them good, nutritious choices, then let them take over.

Avoid the common practice of using dessert as a reward for finishing a meal. Children, like the rest of us, will want dessert whether or not they finish their meal. If they eat past hunger to finish a meal, sweet will still appeal to them, leading to an excess intake of calories. Instead, offer only reasonable options for dessert, and make these available at limited times (e.g., only after dinner, not after lunch, only certain days of the week).

Do not rule out snacking for your children, any more than for yourself. We have all been advised not to snack before meals. Why? "It will spoil your appetite." Great! What could be better than spoiling our appetites, when our appetites are part of why we are an increasingly overweight society? Give your children access to nutritious snacks, and give them free rein to spoil their appetites. In fact, go ahead and join them!

Of Preaching, and Practice

And with regard to joining them, it is in fact important. In diet as in all things, children respond well to role models. The resistance your children may have shown to changes in their diets may relate in part to your own ambivalence and inconsistency. If you adopt and demonstrate a healthful dietary pattern, you become a positive role model.

Be attentive to the messages your kids are receiving about food from other sources. For example, while watching television, your children will be barraged with enticements to eat "junk" food. This exposure is just as important to supervise as media violence.

Be patient, gentle, and compromising, but be firm. If you are like most parents, you would not accept your children smoking in your home just because they want to! It is time to acknowledge that on a population basis, poor dietary habits are actually a bigger threat to our children than tobacco. Once you have solidified your own commitment to eating in a more healthful way, you are quite justified in insisting that your children accompany you. Avoid establishing a pattern of multiple family meal plans. The inconvenience of this will erode your resolve to eating well, even as it excludes your children from the health benefits of better nutrition. This is important; be steadfast! By making good use of several simple strategies, you can make the way to eating well open up to your whole family.

Obstacle/Opportunity 3
Conflicting Messages by "Experts"

To satisfy our seemingly insatiable appetite for diet-related information, the media keep us all constantly apprised of the latest scientific discoveries and "breakthroughs." In the process, you likely have been getting the impression that no two nutrition experts can agree, and no nutrition advice lasts more than a day. Adding to the dangers of this confusion is our receptiveness to it. After all, if we don't know what we should eat—if even the "experts" can't make up their minds—then why not eat whatever we want? This kind of thinking leads many people to give up their efforts at achieving nutritional health. Thus, conflicts in expert opinion, and our willingness to use apparent inconsistency in nutrition information as an excuse, represent a significant obstacle to eating well.

The Then/Now Conflict

Throughout most of human history and prehistory, information about food was limited. People generally knew what was safe, and what was toxic, and they of course knew what they liked. But beyond that, our ancestors were not subject to conflicting food messages. For the most part, people ate what they could—ruled by necessity rather than opinion.

In the modern, industrialized environment, food is as essential for life as ever, while at the same time it is one of the leading contributors

---

News Flash!

We interrupt this program to point out that fruit and vegetables are still good for you! Film at 11.

Now back to our regularly scheduled program...

---

to chronic disease and premature death. This casts food in terms of both "risk" as well as "benefit," and creates intense interest in authoritative guidance. The combination of our interest, extensive ongoing research, and the media's commitment to providing us stories that will attract our attention creates a situation in which nutrition information is a hot commodity. As a result, we are all subject to nutrition news nearly every day, much of it at odds with what we heard yesterday, or will hear tomorrow. Unlike our ancestors, we have nutritional plenty, and thus can choose food based on information, rather than just availability. Thus, misinformation has the potential to lead us astray.

Strategy

There are, of course, differences of opinion among nutrition experts, as there are among the experts in any field. But these differences are generally modest, and all occur within the context of substantial agreement. The nutrition community is nearly universal in its support of a diet rich in grains, fruits, and vegetables, and restricted in saturated fat and processed foods. And the evidence to back up the prevailing view of diet and health is overwhelming. So, confront any apparent conflicts in expert opinion with a clear, strong opinion of your own, and you will be much less subject to confusion. The first strategy, then, is to approach circulating views with a solid understanding of nutrition and health.

Looking for the "New" in "News"

Conflict is interesting, and marketable. The media much prefer conflict to consensus. You can well imagine that a news flash every day for the last forty-five years that fruits and vegetables really do promote health would get a bit dull after a while!

In order to create *news* where relatively little is actually *new*, the media tend to go out of their way to present controversy. If ten thousand scientists agree with what we've known for decades, and one disagrees, which makes for a news story? So, remember that you hear about controversy because controversy sells.

At the Speed of Science

Another way to make yourself impervious to competing expert opinion is to understand that science and research are incremental by design. No one study gives a definitive answer. Rather, each study is designed to contribute a small amount to a large, and slowly growing body of knowledge.

One study about the health effects of antioxidant vitamins, or zinc, or fatty acids does not change everything we knew before. The findings might contribute to the prior understanding, or help alter it slightly. But, again, in the news media, it is the latest and most controversial finding that gets the most attention.

Avoid the Collusion Illusion

Finally, your susceptibility to the threat of competing expert opinion, and your ability to convert this obstacle to good nutritional health into another opportunity, depends in part on you being very candid with yourself. Most of us *know* that french fries and ice cream almost certainly should not be the bulk of our diet. But if experts can't agree on what to eat to promote health, why not eat ice cream, or french fries, or hot dogs until they figure it out? Because so many of us have experienced so must frustration in efforts to eat well, giving up entirely is always tempting, and when experts seem to disagree, it is an invitation to do so.

It is an invitation you should decline! First, with the strategies you are now mastering, you will overcome obstacles that previously frustrated you. Second, with your solid understanding of nutrition and health, you will realize that there is in fact very little disagreement among nutrition experts. In general, if something you hear seems too good to be true, it likely is.

Obstacle/Opportunity 4: Costs, or Perceptions Regarding Costs, of Nutritious Foods

The conventional wisdom is that "healthy" food is expensive food. If you believe that, it may make you reluctant to improve your nutritional health, and thereby be an obstacle.

While there are ways in which eating for health can cost more, there are even more ways in which it can cost less than the typical modern diet. In comparing diets consistent with nutrition guidelines to the "typical" American diet, the American Medical Association has found that the health-promoting dietary pattern costs, on average, $230 less per adult per year. If it can improve your nutritional health while saving money, it represents a golden opportunity!

Strategy

The folklore that eating a healthful diet is costly comes from looking only at individual foods, instead of the overall diet. As noted above, when the costs of the entire diet are considered, eating well costs *less* than eating poorly.

Many "health food" items are expensive. The companies that make specialty products tend to have smaller volume sales than the large commercial food manufacturers. Smaller volume generally means higher prices. This is true of baked goods, snack foods, and cereals.

In addition, vine-ripened produce, and especially organically grown produce, tends to cost more than the alternatives. Here the issues are again volume, as well as production costs, and short shelf-life. But, you get what you pay for. The costlier produce is often more flavorful. If you are concerned about traces of pesticides and other chemicals in your food, then the higher cost of organic produce may be justified for you as well.

But that's where the bad news ends, and the good news begins. Relative to meat and animal products, plant-based foods are generally less expensive. Each time you substitute beans, lentils, or tofu for meat the fiber and nutrient content of the diet goes up, while the fat content and cost go down.

Whole grains are generally inexpensive. By increasing the proportion of your diet based on whole-grain oats, rice, wheat, couscous, or barley, you improve your nutritional health and save money. Butter and cream are expensive; you save money by reducing their levels in your diet. Soda is expensive, and water is better for you; the more you substitute water for soda, the more money you save.

You get the idea. The more you revise your diet closer to the pattern recommended, the more cost savings you will encounter. And by the time you've settled securely on the *way to eat*, you will likely be approximating the savings reported by the AMA.

Obstacle/Opportunity 5
Folklore: Danger of "Skipping" Breakfast

Views about food—what, when, how to eat, and what not to eat—that are passed along most frequently become food folklore and contain both good and bad information.

For example, there is a widespread view that skipping breakfast is in some way harmful. The concept is neither wrong, nor entirely correct. It is often misapplied, doing more harm than good.

The Then/Now Conflict

We, of course, cannot know with certainty exactly what or how our ancestors ate. But we do know a lot about their general dietary pattern. On that basis, we can say with confidence that our ancestors sometimes skipped breakfast! Not because they wanted to, but because they did not always have access to food. Most of the human experience on Earth has been characterized by cycles of feast and famine. There is no breakfast during a famine.

We also know, however, that our ancestors were gatherers as well as hunters, gathering and eating food as they wandered. In this grazing style of eating, there might have been no clearly defined breakfast per se, but there would certainly have been eating in the morning.

In the modern world, those of us with plenty to eat do not experience famine. The closest we come is the fast between dinner and breakfast the next day. It is this "fast" that we "break" in the morning. Our metabolism is well adapted to eating small amounts often, so it does make sense to eat after an overnight fast. But we are also well adapted to tolerate periods without food.

Barbara's Breakfast...

Barbara's breakfast battles were pretty classic. At age thirty-four, she was hoping to lose about 15 lbs, and they weren't coming off. She told me she ate breakfast when she got up at 6:30 A.M., even though she wasn't hungry then—because she had always been told that breakfast was important. She tended to get very hungry about 9 A.M., when she would eat again.

My advice—let the 9 A.M. eating "be" breakfast. And she did. It helped Barbara reorganize her eating throughout the day to coincide with her hunger—and to lose those extra pounds.

Breakfast IS important, but they had no clocks in the Stone Age. It's time to "break" your "fast" when your appetite says so!

Strategy

There is no magical quality to breakfast. The evidence that breakfast is extremely important relates to studies of schoolchildren living in poverty. These children, who are hungry, perform less well in school when they don't eat breakfast than when they do, which is no surprise. But is that information relevant to you or me? Maybe not.

I have known many patients over the years who eat breakfast because they have been told they should. It is folk wisdom most of us have grown up with. But many of these patients are overweight, trying to lose weight, and not necessarily hungry when they first get up in the morning. They nonetheless eat breakfast, because that's the way it's supposed to be!

However, if you eat first thing in the morning even if you are not hungry, you will also eat later in the day when you are hungry. It may be that the calories from a breakfast you feel obligated to eat are simply added to the rest of the day's calories. More total calories may mean more added weight, which is probably not what you want!

Hunger First, Breakfast After

Breakfast is indeed important, but the timing of it is not fixed. Let hunger guide you. If you wake up at 6 A.M., or 7 A.M., and are not hungry

---

It's Ok to "Run," Then Eat...

I realize you won't necessarily be "at leisure" to eat breakfast when-ever you want—but you don't have to be! For years, I've packed up my snack bag, left for work in the morning, and begun eating whenever I got hungry. This typically means a quick bite in-between patient vis-its, followed, of course, by hand-washing!

The only hazard? Getting something stuck between your teeth...

---

until 9 A.M., or 10 A.M., or even 11 A.M., have breakfast then, when you are hungry. There is a big difference between being hungry and unable to eat, and waiting to be hungry before eating.

If you are not hungry first thing in the morning, and delay break-fast until you are hungry, there can be a variety of benefits. By eating later in the morning, your breakfast will probably reduce your appetite for lunch. Your lunch may shrink, which may make a mid-afternoon snack more appealing. A well-timed, well-chosen snack in the afternoon may help you control portion sizes at dinner, or even exercise after work—all of which may lead to better overall nutrition, reduced calorie intake, and weight loss over time. And all due to hav-ing breakfast when you want it, rather than when folk wisdom says you should!

Another advantage of eating breakfast when hungry is that it helps put you in touch with your metabolism. Many of us are so used to eat-ing when we should, or for reasons other than hunger, that we've lost communication with our bodies. Getting back in touch with the basic signals related to hunger, appetite, and satiety is very important in gain-ing control over portion size, the tendency to binge, and total calorie intake. Learn to listen to your body.

Not Just When, but What

Of course, you might be hungry first thing in the morning, in which case you should indeed have breakfast then. The important issue then becomes what you eat, rather than when. Foods that are high in fiber, such as whole-grain cereals, tend to maintain satiety and energy levels much longer than processed foods. So, by choosing a healthful breakfast, you can again set yourself up for portion control and nutritious eating throughout the day.

Recall that for the most part, our relationship with food is too complicated. Adding rules about when to eat a particular meal adds to this complexity. Simplify. Break your overnight fast with a nutritious meal when you feel like it!

Obstacle/Opportunity 6
Folklore: Hazards of Snacking

Most of us have grown up hearing about the hazards of snacking. "Don't eat between meals; you'll spoil your appetite," is right up there with, "Don't talk with your mouth full!" But, the rationale for the first bit of folklore is pretty shaky. As discussed elsewhere, in a society where most of us eat more calories than we need, a bit of appetite "spoiling" wouldn't be so bad!

But there is more to it than that. If snacking is added to meals, it of course adds to the total daily calorie intake, increasing the risk of weight gain. But there is helpful and harmful snacking. The one-size-fits-all rule, "don't snack," causes many of us to avoid eating when hungry, leading to binges and overindulgence

The Then/Now Conflict

Our ancestors almost certainly "snacked"; most hunter-gatherers, and almost all omnivorous animals, do. When one eats low-calorie, highly nutritious foods throughout the day, appetite is held in check, the nutrient profile of the diet tends to be very good, and the relationship with food is simplified in beneficial ways. So snacking is good!

Or at least, snacking *was* good. In modern context, there are two problems with it. The first is that it can interfere with social aspects of eating. If you do not eat with your family at a meal time because you snacked just prior, it can disrupt the gathering. Someone who prepared a meal (perhaps you) may feel hurt when someone else does not join in. So to some extent, we have developed a snacking "prohibition" based on social aspects of eating.

The other problem with modern snacking is the nature of the snacks. Snacking is always good when you are grazing on plants! But our grazing may involve chips, cookies, crackers, and cheese, and can thus add tremendously to our total intake of fat, calories, sugar, and/or salt. So, snacking well is good; snacking badly is bad!

Strategy

By eating well-selected snacks each day, you can avoid excessive hunger and fear of hunger; suppress the tendency to binge eat; reduce insulin release; control appetite; alleviate stress; obtain gratification; and sustain a high energy level. We recommend, in particular, fresh fruit, fresh vegetables (e.g., baby carrots), dried fruit, whole-grain breads, whole-grain crackers, small servings of nuts, and/or nonfat dairy products as particularly beneficial snacks. You can virtually adjust your appetite for meals up or down by the type, quantity, and timing of snacks you choose. Over time, you will work out a regimen that's best for you.

The Fine Art of Spoiling Your Appetite

Because you can control your snacking, and how it relates to your meals, you can easily accommodate the social aspects of eating. If you are eating alone, or don't have any family meals planned, then you may want to shift more of your daily calories from meals to snacks.

If participating in one or more family meals per day, or week, is important to you, you can adjust your snacking downward before those occasions so you can participate fully. Even then, you may benefit from some premeal snacking, to take the edge off your appetite and control any tendency you might otherwise have to overindulge during the meal.

This seems a good time to remind you that multiple strategies for eating well interrelate. For snacking to be beneficial, you need to know what snacks to choose. To have access to healthful snack items, you need to know what to shop for, what to put in your pantry, and how to prepare and transport these items conveniently. For your snacking to fit in well with social aspects of eating, remember to let your family and friends know that you are working to improve your diet, health, and/or weight. If you snack before a meal someone else prepares and don't eat much, they might be hurt. But if you tell them (or yourself if you're the cook!), "It's because this/your food is so good that I snacked a little while ago; otherwise, I wouldn't trust myself," you can avoid hurt feelings and even engage some help as you continue along your new *way to eat*.

For more detailed guidance on how to snack well, see Section IV, Resource 6.

Obstacle/Opportunity 7
Food Categorization or Generalization

Recently, a friend who struggles to control her weight was describing her efforts as we walked together. Her description of dietary restraint, and commitment to regular physical activity, was compelling. Yet despite these efforts, weight control was proving elusive.

At one point in the conversation, she asked if perhaps a whole-grain bagel might be a better choice than an "everything" bagel. The "everything" toppings, including various seeds and sprinkled cheese, on her bagel may have been providing her over two hundred calories more than the "generic" bagel she was using to calculate her daily energy intake!

An excess of two hundred calories a day, unaccounted for, could represent a weight gain of nearly half a pound per week, or twenty-five pounds in a year! What we actually eat, not the names or categories of foods, is what matters in energy balance and weight regulation. And the wide variations in food within any given category in modern society makes accuracy about dietary intake a real challenge. To achieve a realistic estimate of your dietary intake (see Step 3), which is critical in efforts to improve diet and weight, this challenge must be overcome.

The Then/Now Conflict

Familiarity with particular foods was important for our ancestors. Many foods in any given category, such as berries or roots, can vary from health-promoting to poisonous. It was important to know the difference!

The hazards of variation within a category now tend to relate much more often to how we process foods. Not all bread shares any particular nutritional profile, nor do crackers, cereals, soups, or even meat. Food processing, food additives, and creative labeling result in a wide

---

Romeo, Roses, & Ratatouille...

"What's in a name? That which we call a rose, by any other word, would smell as sweet..." says Juliet to Romeo in Shakespeare's *Romeo and Juliet*.

Just as the sweet smell of a rose would still be there no matter what we called it, the nutritional composition of a food may not have anything to do with its name. You can call something a "salad," but if it's mostly bacon bits, croutons, cold cuts, and cheese, rather than fresh greens, it will still be a load of fat and calories! It would probably sound better if Shakespeare said it, but you get the idea!

---

variety of "nutritional profiles" under any given food name. Just as our ancestors needed to know the difference between berries that were safe and berries that might look similar but were toxic, we need to know the actual content of food, not just its name or category, to stick with plans for eating well.

Strategy

In efforts directed at weight control and nutritional health, honesty with yourself is not only the best policy, it is the only policy that works. But the opposite of honesty need not be dishonesty, it may be lack of information or, more bluntly, ignorance. Don't be offended! Ignorance of food composition is nearly universal in modern society, where food is so often drastically altered from its natural state. The ingredient list in some processed foods can read like an encyclopedia entry. But just as "ignorance of the law" does not satisfy a court as a basis for breaking the law, ignorance of actual dietary intake will not satisfy your metabolism. If you take in too many calories, your weight will go up. If you eat too much saturated fat, your cholesterol will rise.

Don't think of food in categories, think of actual foods you eat.

Small miscalculations across a wide range of foods can amount to enormous miscalculations in energy intake, which in turn can undermine weight control efforts, and generate terrible frustration.

What's in a Name?

Fruits and vegetables in their natural state vary within a narrow enough range that worrying about the variation is not productive. The more foods tend to be processed or modified, the more subject they are to within-category variation in nutrient composition. This is true of cereals, breads, pastas, soups, cookies, and snack foods to name a few.

Even more variation is introduced when foods are combined, particularly when processed foods are combined with other processed foods. For example, a "turkey sandwich" combines variable turkey with variable bread, along with variable condiments and variable spread!

Variation in Nutritional Composition Among Foods Sharing the Same Name

The nutrient composition values are approximations derived from the USDA Nutrient Database for Standard Reference, Release 14 (http://www.nal.usda.gov /fnic/cgi-bin/nut_search.pl). Total fat is shown in grams, and in parentheses as calories, and percent of total calories.

Representative Nutritional Variation Implicit in the "Turkey Sandwich" Category:

Nutrient	Turkey Sandwich A	Turkey Sandwich B
	Lean turkey breast, whole-grain bread, lettuce, tomato, mustard	Processed turkey loaf, white bread, provolone, mayonnaise
Total calories	246	613
Total fat	4 grams (36 kcal; 15%)	35 grams (315 kcal; 51%)
Saturated fat	1 gram	14 grams
Sodium	1,627 mg	1,630 mg
Fiber	5 grams	1 gram

— Even All Chocolate Is Not Created Equal! —

It may be especially surprising to learn that even "chocolate" is a whole category of foods, and that choices within this category provide very different nutrition.

The most important distinction to make is between milk chocolate and dark, or bittersweet, chocolate. The fatty acid, or type of fat, found most abundantly in bittersweet chocolate is called *stearic acid*. Although it is a saturated fat, stearic acid does not behave like other saturated fats, and does not raise cholesterol levels. Milk chocolate, however, contains milk fat in addition to the natural "chocolate" fat. Milk fat provides a lot of *palmitic acid*, which *does* raise cholesterol. The bottom line is that dark chocolate is thought to be "heart-healthy," while milk chocolate is not.

In addition to this, milk chocolate generally provides more sugar, and therefore may stimulate appetite more. Eating milk chocolate is thus likely to lead to more fat, more calories, and more potential harm to health than eating dark chocolate.

Our recommendation? If you are a chocolate fan, have dark chocolate in the house, rather than milk chocolate. When you get that irresistible chocolate urge, satisfy it with the dark chocolate. You'll get your chocolate "fix," but with better nutrition, less fat, and fewer calories.

This same sort of substitution works in many food categories, allowing you to eat the type of food you like, while improving your nutrition at the same time. That's a win-win situation if ever there was one.

This type of variation is a recurrent theme throughout our food supply. Even "a cup of coffee" is a category, rather than an actual food item. A six-ounce mug of coffee drunk black provides 3.5 calories; the same mug with a teaspoon of added skim milk provides 5.3 calories; while that mug with two packets of sugar and two tablespoons of Half & Half offers ninety calories!

Thinking Inside the Box

To combat the hazards of food generalizations, you need to understand the basics of healthful eating and to assess your specific dietary intake. Then, you need to decide what changes to make within food categories.

This effort at first requires that you read the details provided in the *Nutrition Facts* on food labels. But the labor-intensive aspect of this strategy doesn't last long. Once you come to know specific foods within given categories that do meet your nutritional standards, you can just stick with them.

Obstacle/Opportunity 8: Food Inattentiveness

Because it would be hard for you to say with certainty what you ate last week, or perhaps even yesterday, tracking dietary intake is very challenging. But it is also important for you to make accurate assessments of your current diet as a basis for knowing what warrants changing.

Some types of foods are particularly easy to overlook. When you have a sandwich, you may not think much about the spread. Salad dressing may not be memorable. You may not have even been paying attention when you grabbed a handful of nuts. The cream cheese spread, slice of cheese, cream sauce, or high-calorie snack that you don't think about may be the reason your weight is going up when you think it should be going down. This "food inattentiveness" is an important potential obstacle to eating well. Conversely, attentiveness to the details of your diet can create great opportunities for improvements.

The Then/Now Conflict

Eating too much, having constant access to high-calorie snack foods, and the availability of complex foods with dressing, spreads, and sauces are all aspects of the modern nutritional environment. Our ancestors faced no such challenges. They ate relatively simple foods, and for the most part, could not overeat if they wanted to. Only an environment in which food is abundantly and constantly available, and in which food preparation is often a commercial rather than personal undertaking, could give rise to food inattentiveness.

Mandy's Mystery...

Mandy, forty-five, was adamant that she was barely eating anything. So her rising weight was a mystery. I was really at a loss: how could someone take in so few calories and still gain weight? Her food diary showed good eating habits and confirmed her low calorie intake. Her blood work was all normal. She even came in with her husband, who confirmed—as a first-hand witness—how little Mandy ate at meal times.

It took a while, but Mandy's mystery was solved. Food inattentiveness! She had three kids and routinely finished the foods they left on their plates. There were occasional donut holes at work, and the occasional candy bar while doing errands. When it was all added up, it came to nearly 400 kcal per day—more than enough reason for weight gain—and a problem that was easily fixed once the mystery was solved!

Strategy

Well, to put it bluntly: be attentive! Our bodies respond to the nutrients and calories we eat, whatever we call them, whether or not we recall them. You may feel you eat very few calories and should be losing weight, or eat very little fat and should be lowering your cholesterol. You may get so frustrated that you actually feel persecuted, as if the rules of energy balance are being unfairly applied to you!

To be fair, you may indeed have a low basal metabolism, and may gain weight at a calorie level that would let others lose weight. But you may be underestimating your intake of calories, or fat, or sugar. This tendency is widespread, so don't be surprised if it affects you.

Looking Over What You've Been Overlooking

Whether or not you complete a full diary of your dietary intake, think in detail about the foods you eat.

Spreads—cream cheese, butter, margarine, mayonnaise—count. Dressings—bleu cheese, creamy Italian, Caesar—count. Sauces count.

And snacks count. Throughout this text, we've recommended snacking—but we've also been quite particular about the kinds of snacks. Nuts are nutrient dense, but also very calorie dense, and are the type of snack that can easily add several hundred calories to your daily intake, and yet be overlooked.

Once you assess how much food inattentiveness you are subject to, you can begin to compensate. Start by factoring in the calories, fat, sugar, and salt of the overlooked items to make a realistic appraisal of your current diet relative to the diet you would like. Then, identify which items you consider most expendable. You might, for example, be willing to take cream, or sugar, out of your coffee. Perhaps instead of eliminating something, you prefer to replace it. But you can only make these kinds of decisions once you've taken a thorough inventory of what you're eating, replacing inattentiveness with awareness.

Obstacle/Opportunity 9
Inability to Interpret Food Labels

Our food supply is rich in highly processed products, often with lengthy ingredient lists, so that no simple assumptions about their nutrient composition can be made based on a "main" ingredient. Much useful information is available on the nutrition label. But chances are, you are not completely secure in your ability to interpret a nutrition label (if you are, then skip this obstacle!).

Strategy

Food label interpretation is addressed in detail in Section IV. In brief, consider reading food labels an important part of the transition to a healthful diet, not an ongoing obligation. Once you come to know which foods, product lines, and brands are consistent with your nutritional goals, you will recognize them at a glance, and won't need to continue reading labels. Whenever a product changes, or you are considering adding something new to your diet, you will once again have cause to call on your label-reading ability. But more and more, you will simply be eating foods you know to be nutritious. Once you get used to the dietary changes you are making, they stop being effort-dependent.

The Food Facts

There are two basic components of nutrition labels: the ingredient list, and the nutrient profile. Here are two examples: labels from Kraft Philadelphia Light Cream Cheese Spread, and Cape Cod Reduced Fat Potato Chips.

Representative food labels, including both nutrition facts, and ingredients.

A) *Kraft Philadelphia Light Cream Cheese Spread*

Nutrition Facts

Serving size 2 tbsp (32g)
Servings about 7

Amount per serving	
Calories 60	Calories from Fat 45

	% Daily Value*
Total Fat 4.5g	7%
Saturated Fat 3g	15%
Cholesterol 15mg	5%
Sodium 150mg	6%
Total Carbohydrate 2g	1%
Dietary Fiber 0g	
Sugars 2g	
Protein 3g	

Vitamin A 8%	•	Vitamin C 0%
Calcium 4%	•	Iron 0%

*Percent Daily Values (DV) are based on a 2,000 calorie diet.

INGREDIENTS: Pasteurized Milk and Cream, Whey, Whey Protein Concentrate, Cheese Culture, Salt, Stabilizers (Xanthan and/or Carob Bean and/or Guar Gums), Lactic Acid, Sorbic Acid as a Preservative, Natural Flavor, Vitamin A Palmitate

Label Reading, 101

The first thing to look for on the ingredient list is how long it is. In general, natural foods have short ingredient lists, and processed foods have longer ones. Note that the potato chips have only three ingredients: potatoes, oil, and salt. Choose foods with short lists, and limit intake of foods with long lists, especially if there are many chemical names.

B) *Cape Cod Reduced Fat Potato Chips*

Nutrition Facts	
Serving size 1 oz. (28g/about 19 chips)	
Servings per container 5	

Amount per serving	
Calories 130	Calories from Fat 50

	% Daily Value
Total Fat 6g	**9%**
Saturated Fat 2g	**3%**
Polyunsaturated Fat 2g	
Monounsaturated Fat 3.5g	
Cholesterol 0mg	**0%**
Sodium 110mg	**5%**
Total Carbohydrate 18g	**6%**
Dietary Fiber 1g	**4%**
Sugars Less than 1g	
Protein 2g	

Vitamin A 0%	•	Vitamin C 10%	
Calcium 0%	•	Iron 2%	

• Percent Daily Values (DV) are based on a 2,000 calorie diet. Your daily values may be higher or lower depending on your calorie needs:

	Calories	2,000	2,500
Total Fat	Less than	65g	80g
Sat Fat	Less than	20g	25g
Cholesterol	Less than	300mg	300mg
Sodium	Less than	2,400mg	2,400mg
Total Carbohydrate		300g	375g
Dietary Fiber		25g	30g

Calories per gram:
Fat 9 • Carbohydrate 4 • Protein 4

The fat content has been reduced from 10 grams for regular potato chips to 6 grams per serving.

INGREDIENTS: Potatoes, Canola Oil, and Salt

There are, however, two exceptions of note. First, a product with many varieties of grains, such as a multigrain bread or a veggie burger, may have a relatively long list of ingredients, all of which are good for you. Also, foods fortified with many vitamins and minerals will include them all in the ingredient list; these are not harmful, and may be beneficial. So be prepared to make some exceptions.

The next thing to look for on the ingredient list is additions in particular categories, such as fat, sugar, or sodium. Look for oils, and avoid tropical oils (palm kernel oil, coconut oil), and "partially hydrogenated" oils (usually soybean or cottonseed oils; the label will generally state "may contain one or more of the following partially hydrogenated oils: soybean, and/or cottonseed, and/or…"). Also, avoid cream, as it is a concentrated source of saturated fat. The cream cheese lists cream among the first ingredients. Note that all ingredients are listed in order of abundance, so the food is made up mostly of the ingredients that come early on the list.

Look for added sugars in the form of sugar, fructose, or corn syrup. Look for added sodium in the form of salt, but also as sodium bicarbonate, and other sodium-containing compounds. Limit your intake of foods with these added items.

Making Sense of the "Percent Daily Value"

As for the *Nutrition Facts*, there are some basics that tell you most of what you need to know. Look at the calories per serving size, then look at the calories from fat per serving size. If the fat calories are more than 30 percent of the total, consider the item relatively high in fat, because it has more fat than you want for your overall diet. This gets a little confusing, because the percent of calories from fat in the serving is different from the "percent daily value" shown on the nutrition label. The percent daily value tells you what percentage of total daily calories, usually set at two thousand, that should come from any particular class of nutrient, such as fat, are provided in a serving of the food you're eating.

To make sense out of this, consider that you eat a 2,000 kcal per day diet. To keep your fat intake less than 30 percent of calories, no more than 600 daily calories should come from fat (0.3 X 2,000). This is about 65 grams of fat per day. The grams of fat in a serving are divided by those 65 grams, then multiplied by 100, to give the percent daily value. If a serving of some food, such as oil, is 100 kcal, and all of them are from fat, this would be about 11 grams of fat. Dividing those 11 grams by 65, then multiplying by 100, gives 17 percent. This is the "percent daily value" for fat in a serving of this food. The serving of oil provides about 17 percent of the fat you should eat in a day.

But the percent of calories from fat in the serving is much simpler: it's 100 percent if all of the calories are from fat. A serving of cream cheese provides 60 kcal, and 45 of these are from fat. The percent of calories from fat in a serving is therefore (45/60) X (100), or 75 percent. Since this is way over the recommended upper limit of 30 percent, the cream cheese should be considered a high-fat food, which makes sense since cream is one of the primary ingredients. The potato chips provide 130 kcal per serving, and 50 of these are from fat. The percent of calories per serving from fat is therefore (50/130) X (100), or 38 percent. So, even though these are fat-reduced potato chips, they still provide more fat than you want on average in your diet. This makes them a relatively high-fat food, too. After all, if all of the foods you eat, even the "fat-reduced" foods, provide a higher percentage of fat than you want in your diet overall, your diet overall will, of course, contain more fat than you want!

Then, look for fiber. Try to choose foods that provide 2 or more grams of fiber per 100 calories (kcal). These are foods that generally contain natural grains, beans, or vegetables.

If you think in terms of a 100 kcal serving size, you can simply try to pick products with less than 30 fat calories (about 3 grams of fat), and 2 or more grams of fiber. You can, of course, make exceptions, but as a general rule, this approach will guide you toward healthful eating. Neither the cream cheese nor the potato chips makes the cut if you apply this "1-2-3 rule" (1 serving size of 100 kcal; 2 or more grams of fiber; 3 or less grams of fat).

Obstacle/Opportunity 10
Sabotage, Well-Meaning & Otherwise

If you have ever tried to lose weight, or to change your diet to improve your health, you have almost certainly encountered "diet sabotage." You may or may not have recognized it at the time.

If you are overweight and your friends tell you you are not, "So go ahead and have another slice of pizza...," if your significant other brings home the very foods you are trying to resist, if a friend or family member asks, "Are you feeling all right? Your face is so thin..." as you struggle to shed excess pounds, it's diet sabotage, and it's very widespread.

Clothing Conspiracy...

Men's clothes are typically measured in a pretty standard way. But apparently the sizing of women's clothing is more variable. I have heard it suggested that the actual size of a "size 8" dress has *increased* over time! The idea seems to be to make you feel good by letting you believe you fit into the same size clothes you did years ago. But if what I've heard is true, a "size 8" ain't what it used to be—and what that tends to imply is, neither are we! (*With thanks to Meghan O'Connell, MPH, for a keen observation.*)

It may be nice to still fit into your old size clothes, but you know whether or not that actually makes sense. There is no shame in being overweight, so there's no harm in admitting it.

Being honest while being understanding—that's the way!

The reasons for it are diverse. You may seem to be struggling, and your friends or family may genuinely want to help you feel better about yourself. Sometimes, if you are succeeding with dietary change, you make someone who is not succeeding feel badly about themselves; it helps them feel OK if you fail, too. Most of the sabotage is not malicious, and much of it is not even conscious. But it can represent a considerable obstacle to nutritional health unless you know it for what it is, and deal with it well.

Strategy

First, recognize diet sabotage when it's happening. To be blunt, you know whether or not you are too fat! You also know whether your blood pressure, blood sugar, or cholesterol is too high. If you don't know these things, you probably should. In terms of the medical tests, you will need your doctor's help. The weight you can assess on your own. Use a scale you trust, and compare your weight to what you want it to be. Take a look at yourself, from all views, in a full-length mirror, wearing only your skin. You'll know whether your friends who tell you not to lose weight are being honest or not. Try on some clothes that fit you well when you are/were at your preferred weight. These clothes won't fib, even if your friends and family do.

Once you have done your reality check, assess the sources and extent of diet sabotage you are encountering. Be sure to do this unemotionally, and avoid getting angry at anyone; remember that little if any of the sabotage is intentional or malicious. You may even have committed some yourself!

Then, try to figure out the likely reasons for the sabotage. You may or may not be able to do this in every case, and it may not be necessary. It's most important if the sabotage is coming from someone very close to you, especially your significant other.

Catching "Saboteurs" with Honey

The one strategy that will work well most of the time is simply to make a direct request for help. Say to whomever is sabotaging your efforts at nutritional health something like, "I wanted you to know I'm working on improving my diet/health/weight, and it's quite challenging. I was hoping you could help me." Then go on to address the relevant issues: ask not to be offered food, or to be coaxed, or flattered. Be gentle, but firm. If it seems appropriate, you might ask the person you are addressing to join you in your pursuit of better eating, and offer to support their efforts as they support yours.

In some cases, the conversation may get a little more complicated. If nervousness, jealousy, or envy are involved, you may need to address these things. You may need to reassure an uneasy spouse or significant other. Use your good judgement, and you will almost certainly find these discussions productive and helpful.

Simply by recognizing and understanding diet sabotage, you remove it as an obstacle. But if you go further, the people formerly undermining your pursuit of healthful eating may speed you on your way, or even join you.

The Right Words for Help That Are…Helpful

Asking for help is a good first step toward preventing sabotage. But if you are not clear about the kind of help you need, you can't be sure of the kind of help you'll get. Consider whether you want moral support, encouragement, guidance, or help with discipline. Will you appreciate it, or resent it, if a friend uses guilt or shame to try and keep you on track? Do you want just positive feedback when you do well, just negative feedback when you do not so well, or both? Once you've decided what kind of help you want, ask for it very specifically.

Obstacle/Opportunity 11
Social "Normalization" of Being Overweight

"Normal" is in the eyes of society or culture just as "beauty" is in the eyes of the beholder. One of the standard ways of deciding what is or is not "normal," appropriate, acceptable, or ideal in any society is the so-called *"bell curve."* The "bell curve" represents the range of any particular characteristic, such as IQ, within which most of the population falls. If you are near the middle of the bell curve, you are more or less "average" with regard to whatever is being measured. If you are way out to either side, you have more or less of the particular characteristic than most people in the population.

With regard to weight, your position in the population bell curve may move up, or down, as your weight moves up or down. But the whole curve is also moving! The United States gets a little more overweight each year. As a result, the mean, or average, weights for the population keep moving up. If your weight is above average but stays stable over time, the average may well catch up to you!

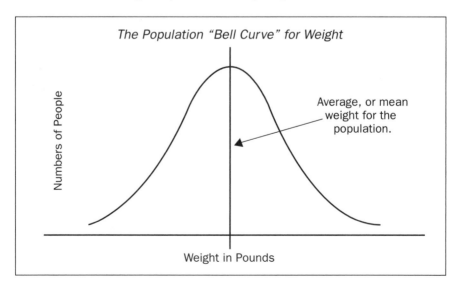

The Population "Bell Curve" for Weight

Numbers of People

Average, or mean weight for the population.

Weight in Pounds

What this means is that looking around, you will see more and more overweight people until, or unless, we find ways to stop this trend. The more overweight those around you are, the less overweight you are in comparison.

Being overweight is not the fault of the individual, and should not be treated as if it were. But being overweight does have health consequences. Even if those around you are heavier than you are, your weight can still affect your health. Social normalization of being overweight refers to moving up the threshold for desirable weight as the population weight rises. Doing so might be good if it helps remove some of the inappropriate stigma attached to being overweight. But it ignores the link between weight and health, which does not depend on social conventions.

The Then/Now Conflict

Perceptions of desirable weight have changed over time. We cannot know what our prehistoric ancestors found attractive, but chances are if they ever experienced being overweight, they liked it. Why wouldn't they? Most cultures seem to admire traits that are rare or difficult to attain, and in the primitive world, being overweight would be both.

We have good evidence from more recent history that heavier was preferred to thinner. If the subjects of those Renaissance paintings of nude women represent the beauties of their day, it is clear that more flesh was preferred to less. This is true today, as well, in many cultures.

Our own societal standards of weight and attractiveness are in flux. We clearly admire thinness, as represented by our models and movie stars. But we also see more and more overweight people in our daily lives, and as a result may be slowly ratcheting up our perception of what "real" overweight is.

Strategy

First, separate considerations of health and physical attractiveness. You can be very attractive, but have high cholesterol, high blood pressure, or diabetes. If you do, you are probably interested in using nutrition to improve your health and reduce your long-term risk. If you concentrate on eating well and being active, you can let your weight take care of itself.

Even so, it is useful to have some guidelines to consider as you gauge your weight, and its relationship to health. The National Institutes of Health (NIH) have offered some useful guidance here. Based on very extensive data, they have defined being overweight as a body mass index, or BMI, of 25 or higher. Your BMI is your weight in kilograms, divided by your height in meters squared. (A kilogram is 2.2 pounds, and a meter is just about 39 inches.) BMI is the standard measure of weight used by professionals.

The fact that a BMI above 25 is associated with increased risk of chronic illness, such as heart disease and cancer, will not change just because being overweight becomes more and more common in the U.S. The definition of overweight set by the NIH is not based on fashion, prejudice, or social convention, but on the fact that there is increased risk of adverse health effects of weight above this threshold.

The Ways Weight Does, and Doesn't, Matter

First, we believe that being overweight is *not* a reason to feel badly about yourself. For some of us, seeing others who are as, or even more, overweight than we are helps us feel better. Feeling better is good, but there is also the risk that we will all lose our motivation for weight control because everyone else's weight keeps going up! Keeping your body mass index near the levels associated with optimal health is important, and entirely independent of what everyone else's BMI happens to be. What you need to work toward—and it can be quite challenging—is to balance an honest and realistic assessment of your weight relative to your health, without becoming preoccupied with weight as a primary goal, or beating up on yourself!

Obstacle/Opportunity 12
Starting Tomorrow: The Scarlett O'Hara Syndrome

You've almost certainly been there. You make a decision about improving your diet for health and/or weight control. And then, something calls out to you: a slice of pizza, french fries, chocolate cake. And you give in. Then, feeling as if the "damage" has been done, you say, "I'll diet tomorrow." And, since you'll need to "sacrifice" tomorrow, you decide to indulge today.

This approach can lead to cycles of indulgence and deprivation, or to procrastination, either of which can be an obstacle to eating well.

Strategy

The strategy for avoiding the Scarlett O'Hara Syndrome has five basic components. *First,* let tomorrow be today. *Second,* improve your diet at your pace, and accept every improvement you make as a success in its own right. *Third,* never go "on" a diet—simply improve your dietary pattern. *Fourth,* expect and accept the occasional craving, and the occasional lapse in your eating plan; this is not failure. And *fifth,* be forgiving of yourself, even as you exercise restraint.

No Time Like the Present

Let tomorrow be today. As with so much else in nutritional health, this simple strategy depends on many others, all of which you are now learning. If you believe you need to go "on" a diet that will make you hungry and miserable, any rational person would want to put it off as long as possible!

But if instead you decide that you want the benefits of a healthful diet and decide to go after them, there is no reason not to start right now! Take just one step, then follow it with more. No need to suffer; just a need to get started toward a more healthful lifestyle and way of eating. With this in mind, why wait? Start today.

Go at your own pace, and accept each step you take as success. Each new strategy you apply to your diet and health will support many other strategies. Before you know it, even if you are only trying to make small changes, your diet will start to improve itself!

Stay Off the "On & Off"

Remember that if you go "on" a diet that is not manageable or consistent with health, over a lifetime you will inevitably go back "off," and when you do, you will lose whatever you've gained (or gain back whatever you've lost!). Don't ever go "on" a diet again. Eat well. That's different.

As you do begin to improve your dietary pattern, keep in mind that you are not a robot. You will have good days and bad, good moods and bad. Accept that what makes each of us unique also makes all of

---

If You Lapse, It Means...

You are human! Welcome to the family!

---

us susceptible to occasional lapses. You will get better and better at preventing and controlling lapses over time. But if and when they do occur, forgive yourself, and look ahead rather than back. If you are traveling and get one flat tire, it's not a good reason to puncture the other three! So don't use the occasional lapse as a reason to abandon your commitment to more healthful eating altogether.

The Success in Trying
When you delay making improvements in your diet, you may be doing it because you are afraid of failing. But look at it this way: making the commitment is already success! You are trying: good for you!

Think of what you would tell someone you love if they "lapsed" and you were comforting them. Then tell it to yourself—it's all true! Does an occasional misstep mean you're not still headed where you want to go? Of course not! Be forgiving, be committed, and be on your way—today!

Obstacle/Opportunity 13
The Burden of Nutritional "Virtue"
People who are already eating well, and/or are thin and fit, may feel proud, which is not necessarily bad. But they may display this pride by "looking down" on those of us working hard to improve our diets, or to control our weight. If you encounter this, you may feel sorry for yourself. This is an obstacle to making improvements in your nutritional health because it can reduce your self-efficacy.

The opposite is also true. If you are innocently trying to improve your own diet, you may inadvertently make others feel threatened, or bad, because your good effort may make their diet look worse. So, as you try to improve your diet, others may actually resent you. This can exert a strong influence, and represent an obstacle as you try to establish a healthful way of eating.

Finally, if you eat with a group that seems blissfully unconcerned about what they eat, while you work on a healthful diet, you may feel like the nutritional misfit or Goody Two-shoes of the group! This, too, can undermine your commitment to good eating habits.

Together, these potential obstacles are the burden of seeing eating well as a "virtue," rather than a lifestyle choice. With understanding, you can convert these obstacles into opportunities for improving your diet, gaining support, and possibly helping others into the bargain!

Strategy

As you set off on your way to more healthful eating, do not be bothered by the fact that you may see others who are farther along than you. If you modify your diet to promote your health, well-being, weight control, and contentment, is that any less good just because someone else has already done the same thing? Of course not.

Now, what if someone up ahead looks back along the way with an, "Eat my dust!" expression on their face? You have two good options. Ignore them, or enlist their help. You can enlist their help quite simply by addressing the obvious: they are accomplishing something you want to accomplish. Tell them: "I really like the way you eat," or, "You sure do a great job controlling your weight, you look great," and "I'm trying to get there too. Do you have any pointers? I would love advice from someone doing so well."

Everyone likes a well-placed compliment, and you just gave one! You can make the person who's been your "burden" feel good, and get them to help you! Talk about converting an obstacle into opportunity!

On the other hand, if someone you don't particularly care for or know well is flaunting their nutritional virtue at you, ignore them. They may be ahead of you, but so what? You are headed in the right direction for your health and well-being—that's what counts.

Before leaving this topic, let's put the shoe on the other foot, so to speak. As you start to make progress along the way, you will be the one out ahead to many others. And they may see your success as their failure! If they do, they may resent you, or even try to sabotage your efforts. You can prevent this, and help them at the same time.

As you begin improving your dietary pattern, let the people you care most about know what you're up to, and enlist their help. At the same time, offer to help them—sharing your strategies and insights. You can let them know that getting there isn't exactly a piece of cake, and that you weren't just born nutritionally virtuous! You worked at it, and it paid off; they can do the same. The more we share skills and strategies, the more we can support one another, and the more we'll all succeed. On this trip, the more, the merrier!

Finally, don't feel "left out" if you eat with a group that does not choose to join you. Eating well is an important lifestyle choice you are entitled to make. You don't need to be the same religion, or have all the same political views as your friends; you don't need to eat like them, either.

Obstacle/Opportunity 14
Time Constraints That Limit Physical Activity

Eating well and being physically active are two halves of a single, healthy lifestyle. They naturally go together. But social factors are among the many reasons it's difficult to be physically active. Work days, whether outside of home or at home, are long and tiring. Schedules are hectic. If you have small children, their needs fill up every spare minute.

Yet, while exhausting, for most of us our days are also sedentary. We work hard, but not *physically*. We exert ourselves, but without exerting our muscles or conditioning our hearts. This is because the same technology driving the hectic pace of our lives also replaces the work of our muscles much of the time.

As a result, you may be left feeling you simply cannot find the time to be physically active. This matters, because trying to promote your health or control your weight with nutrition but no physical activity is like trying to run on one leg rather than two. Physical activity is an important contributor to the utilization of calories, and therefore to energy balance. It influences metabolism in muscles, the use of glucose and the levels of insulin, and even basal metabolic rate. So not finding time to be physically active has the potential to be an important obstacle.

The Then/Now Conflict

The very things that make us physically inactive—our day to day obligations—are what made our ancestors, both in the distant and recent past, physically active. Before remote controls, electric appliances, or for that matter electricity, all daily chores depended on the work of muscles. The best our predecessors could do, before the Industrial Revolution, was try to get the muscles of animals to replace their own from time to time. But living required physical activity, at a pretty high level, all the time. Our ancestors were not more energetic than we are, not more self-disciplined, and certainly didn't have willpower that we lack. Rather, they simply found it as difficult to be physically inactive as we find it to be physically active!

Strategy

How can you take the very demands on your schedule that make physical activity elusive, and use them to be more physically active?

First, take advantage of the activities you need to do to get physical activity into your day. Do you need to communicate with colleagues at work? Walk to them instead of using the intercom; gain back the little bit of time it takes by being more energetic and alert. Do you need to go up several stories to an office? Take the stairs instead of the elevator. Do you drive to work? Consider parking as far from the building as possible. Better still, think about walking or biking to work if practical for you.

Do you need to shop? Park far from the entrance, and do some extra walking once inside; go up and down every aisle, even if you don't really need to. Do you have housework to do? Put on music, and put a little extra zing into it! If you have yard work to do, use simple tools and your muscles instead of power tools, like leaf and snow blowers, that take away your opportunity for some health-promoting activity.

If you have small children and a significant other, you may be able to work out a schedule that lets you both get in some physical activity. You can, for example, alternate days so that one of you gets to exercise as the other watches the kids. Or take turns on the same day. Or find an activity you can do with your kids, either involving them actively if they are big enough, or just taking them along if they are very little (e.g., placing a child in a back-pack child seat while you go for a walk).

An Ounce of Prevention, on the Go...

I have more than twenty people working with and for me at the Yale Prevention Research Center. It seemed only appropriate that we really practice what we preach, so we've carved out thirty minutes of every day for a group walk—indoors when the weather is bad, outdoors when it's good. My job, as the "boss," is to protect that time and not let anything else be scheduled during *walk time*. I'm confident that this ounce of investment will yield a pound of return—perhaps quite literally if it helps the staff with weight control, but figuratively for sure, by contributing to energy, alertness, fitness, and productivity.

I invite, and challenge, you other "bosses" out there to make this same investment!

Consider turning up your stereo, and dancing with the whole family (we've tested this approach right down to our two-year-old; it works!).

Use your social connections to help you be more active rather than less. Perhaps you can find a group at work that would be willing to walk together at lunchtime. Maybe you can start a walking group in your neighborhood or place of worship. As with eating well, the benefits of physical activity are best shared.

The recommended activity level is at least thirty minutes of moderate activity, such as walking briskly, on most days of the week. But those thirty minutes do not need to occur together; they can add up over the course of the day. So, add activity into your day in small doses wherever you can. If you want additional benefits, consider exercising as well, although physical activity does not need to be in the form of "exercise" to be beneficial. Perhaps you can get up a little bit early and "work out" in the morning; you may find having a treadmill, or Nordic Track, or even aerobic video at home helps you to make the most out of a limited time for exercise. You may find there are particular advantages in being physically active at the end of the workday, but that being hungry makes this difficult. Combine a nutritious, late afternoon snack with after-work exercise for multiple benefits.

As with efforts to improve diet, efforts to work more physical activity into your routine will be more successful if supported by others. Tell your friends, family, employer, or coworkers what you are trying to do. Ask for their help and support, and offer them yours. Social factors can make physical activity difficult, but social factors can also be used to make physical activity more accessible, more convenient, and more enjoyable.

Obstacle/Opportunity 15
Use of Food as Basis for Social Gatherings

If, in your social group, the food that people share is not consistent with your dietary goals, socializing can become an obstacle to eating well. Perhaps, in the past, you've abandoned your efforts to eat well in order to fit in. But you should not need to make a choice between your health and sharing important (or everyday) occasions with the people in your life. By knowing how to handle the challenges of food in social settings, this can become one more opportunity to continue on your way to dietary health, and possibly bring some others along.

The Then/Now Conflict

Food has almost certainly been a fundamental aspect of human interaction throughout all of history. But as with all else in the relationship between humans and food, the implications of food in social gatherings have changed. For our ancestors, the amount of food they could get was limiting, they therefore simply could not "feast" to excess.

We are naturally inclined to continue using food as the basis for our social gatherings, but in modern context, the limits must be imposed by us. We either need to limit the amount of socializing we do, or limit how much, and control what, we eat when we gather.

If we do neither of these things, we are likely to eat more than we should, and probably, of the very foods we should be limiting the most.

Strategy

There are almost as many ways to handle the challenge of food in social settings, as there are ways and reasons to gather. Consider these examples, and assess the social gatherings of importance in your life. Then you decide what strategies are best suited to your needs.

Becoming Atypical

The average diet in the U.S. provides too many calories, too much total fat, too much salt, too little fiber, and too few fruits, vegetables, and grains for optimal health and weight control. If your diet has been a "typical" American diet, then your usual eating pattern has not been ideal. If, on top of that, you tend to indulge somewhat on special occasions (and who doesn't!), it could be the proverbial "last straw," leading to weight gain, or elevated cholesterol, or some other diet-related health problem.

So, the first strategy in preventing social gatherings from compromising your dietary pattern is simply to improve the baseline. In other words, eat well most of the time. If your usual eating habits are good, you gain a whole host of defenses against the potential harm of less healthful eating when you gather, and might well be able to "afford" an occasional indulgence.

What you will tend to find as you grow accustomed to eating well is that even at social gatherings you naturally tend to choose the dishes most supportive of nutritional health. It has probably sneaked up on you, but it's happened: you eat well even when you're not trying!

No Way but the Way

And there is more. In order to eat well most of the time, you need knowledge of what to buy, what to keep in your pantry, what and how to cook. As this knowledge accumulates over time, it too starts to become just the way things are. So, when you are responsible for the social gathering, or for contributing something to it, what you make will tend to be consistent with your healthful pattern of eating. And this doesn't mean the food won't be festive. By substituting ingredients and adapting some of your favorite recipes (see Section IV), you will find that you can prepare many of the dishes you like best, preserving their taste and presentation, and improving the nutrition.

Leaving a Little Appetite at Home

If you are planning to attend a social gathering where you know few foods or dishes will be available that suit your eating habits, you can do the obvious thing: eat ahead of time. You don't need to eat until full,

---

Dietitian Chronicles...

Rosa, forty-three, was terrified of the holiday season. She was struggling to control her weight and her blood pressure, and she *always* gained weight between Thanksgiving and New Year's.

We focused first on some general improvements in her overall diet and activity pattern that she was prepared to make; in other words, getting her started on the *way*. Then we focused on how to combine just a bit of restraint with holiday cheer. The result? Stable weight during the holidays, sure and steady weight loss after. And blood pressure that's now normal! And, because Rosa told her friends and family what she was up to, she has a sister and two cousins as companions—and they are doing just as well! Happy holidays? You bet!

---

and you can keep enough of an appetite to be sociable. But an apple on the way, for example, may help you balance being sociable with being reasonable and restrained.

Your Group, in Motion

You can help move your group toward more healthful eating by setting an example, as well as asking for support. You probably don't want to preach, but there is no harm in being enthusiastic. Suggest to the people you gather with often that you share healthful recipes. Or, get really radical—put a little motion in your social occasions. Maybe your group likes walking or some group sport like volleyball or softball. And if it's an indoor gathering, perhaps you can make a little floor space and dance. Dancing, too, has a long and proud tradition in human gatherings, and it makes a great physical activity—cleverly disguised as fun!

Your Necessity, Your Inventiveness

As noted above, there is no way we can anticipate all of the social gatherings that matter to you—unless you start inviting us to join you! (We'd be honored, but don't feel obligated.) So you will need to be creative.

Think about the groups you eat with, and your role in them. Think about the influence socializing has on your overall dietary pattern, good, bad, or neutral. Weave together the strategies that match these occasions in your life. By doing so, you can blend the pleasure of good company with the health benefits of good eating. And if, as many people do on special occasions, you raise a toast "to health," you'll be well on your way to getting what you ask for!

Step 5:

Traverse the Maze of Food for Mood

THROUGHOUT MOST OF history, our relationship with food was fairly simple: having enough to eat was good. It made sense, under these circumstances, that eating would be recognized as pleasurable and rewarding. It also makes sense that the body systems that register pleasure and gratification would be responsive to food. As a result, our moods and mental health have many built-in connections to the things that we eat. We are, in other words, "hard wired" to be affected emotionally by food.

As a result, our relationship with food now tends to be complicated. Food is a reliable, convenient source of pleasure. In fact, some foods are so intensely pleasurable that their effects on mood can mimic those of mood-enhancing medication. Yet food can also make us pretty unhappy, as the source of weight control or health problems.

Food makes a good reward, and often a good punishment as well. The "psychology" and "neuro-chemistry" of food, and the effects of food on mood, constitute an array of obstacles to eating well. Like the obstacles in other categories, these can be converted into opportunities:

1) Being "Blown Away"

2) Food as Mood Enhancer

3) Food for Pleasure

4) Food as Self-punishment

5) Night-eating Disorder

6) Nutrition Nostalgia

7) Premenstrual Syndrome

8) Seasonal Affective Disorder

9) Stress

Obstacle/Opportunity 1: Being "Blown Away"

Trying to do something over and over and not succeeding is worse than frustrating. After a while, it takes away your belief that you can do it. In behavior change science, this is being *"blown away."*

Often the psychological scars from years of trying to control weight, for example, are quite deep. Your self-esteem may be lower than it should be if you are not already eating as you want to, or weighing what you want to. Low self-esteem can undermine your ability to change, or your self-efficacy.

Strategy

Quite simply: forgive yourself. This entire book is devoted to the concept that eating well in the modern world cannot just happen because you want it to.

It is one thing to be convinced of this; it is quite another to feel it. We are asking you to feel it: you did not fail.

Getting Out of Your Own Way

With the right skills and strategies, you can improve your diet, your health, and your weight. But doing so is not magic, and it's not easy. It is manageable, and it is extremely rewarding. But it starts with some effort. And that effort might be too much if you are carrying the burden of past "failures" that you have not set down.

It may sound odd, but if you want to be on your way to dietary health and weight control, then you must remove from the path in front of you...your former self! Ask politely, or if necessary, give a good hard shove, but get that person who feels as if they've failed out of your way! You cannot carry them and do what needs to be done. Understanding that they never had a chance, because they simply did not know what you now know, should help you realize that it's time for you to take over.

Don't Let This Happen to You...

Loretta, seventy-one, is one of my all-time favorite patients (I realize docs shouldn't have favorite patients, so I'll count on you not to tell!). She is wonderful—sweet, intelligent, interesting. And I'm not the only one who thinks so. She has an adoring husband, loving children and grandchildren, and devoted friends.

But unfortunately, Loretta tends to think of herself as fat. True, since we started working together, she's lost more than fifteen pounds, and has kept the weight off for years. But she's spent just a bit too long being overweight and blaming herself for it. She understands now that she was not to blame, and that she did not fail. But understanding it, and feeling it, aren't quite the same. And I don't think she feels it.

I'm still trying to help Loretta feel the truth. But removing "scars" is tough, and that's what we're up against. My advice to you—avoid these battle scars in the first place. Self-recrimination is *not* a step along the *way to eat*, it's a pot-hole; step around it!

So, it's not just what you ate yesterday or eat today that influences your mood. Your relationship with food over the course of your lifetime gets incorporated into your self-image. What you ate ten years ago could be part of why you felt discouraged yesterday. It's time to start today, and look toward tomorrow. This time, you know the *way*.

Obstacle/Opportunity 2: Food as Mood Enhancer

The influence of food on mood extends beyond the familiar associations with the pleasures of eating and gatherings with loved ones and friends. There is a very direct connection between eating pattern and the brain chemicals that regulate mood.

The brain chemicals that enable our brain cells to communicate with one another are called *neurotransmitters*. While many of these are involved in the regulation of mood, *serotonin* is among the most important. Antidepressants, such as Prozac (fluoxetine), or the herb St. John's Wort, work by raising serotonin levels in the brain.

A Glass of Warm Milk

The time-honored practice of drinking warm milk before sleep has a basis in science; tryptophan is fairly abundant in milk, so drinking milk can help make you sleepy by raising brain serotonin levels! Tryptophan is also relatively abundant in meat and fish.

The amino acid *tryptophan* is a key building block, or precursor, for serotonin. When a supply of tryptophan reaches the brain, serotonin levels go up, generally enhancing mood, and inducing a relaxed state.

Eating processed carbohydrate triggers an insulin release. Insulin causes many other amino acids to be taken up by muscle cells, leaving a "surplus" of tryptophan in the blood. The level of tryptophan that enters the brain is determined in large part by its competition with other amino acids. If lots of other amino acids get to the blood supply of the brain, less tryptophan gets in. If there are few other amino acids around, the brain takes up more tryptophan. So, insulin release causes more tryptophan to get into the brain by removing the competition.

The more tryptophan enters the brain, the more serotonin is produced. This brings the story full circle: eating processed carbohydrate leads to mood enhancement through the effects on brain serotonin levels. There is reason to believe that this "positive reinforcement" can lead to overeating.

The Then/Now Conflict

In a world where getting enough to eat was always a challenge, a plentiful food supply would confer a sense of security, comfort, and contentment. It may be the by-product of these reactions among our ancestors, over countless generations, which ultimately left its imprint on us. This by-product is a response to foods that directly influences brain chemistry, altering mood.

Strategy

As with so many of the potential barriers to eating well, the conversion of this one from obstacle to opportunity begins quite simply by knowing it is there. Food does affect mood. The way we eat affects our brain sero-tonin levels. The influence is normal, predictable, and controllable.

Feeling Good, without Doing Bad

The strategies for meeting this challenge are directed at obtaining the mood-enhancing benefits of food, without overeating.

Serotonin levels can be kept at consistent levels if enough tryptophan gets to the brain. This can be achieved if dietary protein intake is mod-erate and consistent, and if insulin levels are similarly moderate and consistent. The dietary pattern we recommend will get the job done.

Snacking on appropriate foods is a good start. Eating regularly helps to control insulin levels. Our current understanding suggests that avoid-ance of insulin surges prevents the "carbohydrate craving" that large fluctuations in tryptophan delivery to the brain can otherwise cause.

Eat complex carbohydrate as the mainstay in your diet. Whole grains, beans, legumes, fruits, and vegetables are generally rich in fiber, both sol-uble and insoluble. Soluble fiber is especially important in promoting a slow and steady release of glucose into the blood stream, which in turn evokes a moderate insulin response. The result is consistent delivery of tryptophan to the brain, and a consistent mood-enhancing benefit of food, rather than a sudden peak, followed by an abrupt crash.

The same dietary pattern that is good for your health is good for your mood. Eat well, feel well—that's the way to go!

Obstacle/Opportunity 3: Food for Pleasure

Pleasurable effects of eating related to taste, a sense of fullness (satiety), comfort, security, and even the texture of foods cause some of us to overeat total calories, fat, or sugar, and to use food to relieve stress or anxiety, or simply to make ourselves feel good.

Strategy

Be aware that, in general, the foods that make us feel especially good when we eat them are the foods our ancestors needed most, not neces-sarily the foods we need the most! You cannot count on the pleasure you get from eating to guide you to a healthful dietary pattern. In fact, if not kept in check, the pleasure response to food will lead to excess intake of fat and sugar especially. So, you need to take some control of this situation—don't let a Neanderthal tell you what to eat!

There are several key components to managing the pleasure responses to food. One is to know what constitutes a healthful diet, and to let this guide your dietary choices. By following the lead of knowledge, you will be able to tell when pleasure is trying to take you somewhere knowledge says you should not go.

Knowledge of what nutrients are in which foods is also important. By choosing foods that do not contain large amounts of added sugar or fat, you can reduce the levels of your usual intake. You can also protect yourself against "hidden" ingredients often added to processed foods. Many foods you would not expect to contain fat, or sugar, or salt, do. These ingredients affect your pleasure response, whether or not you know they are there.

Staying Out of "Pleasure Debt"

Another important consideration is to avoid developing a large "pleasure debt," a lack of fun or relaxation, that only food will fix. There are two ways of doing this. One is to use food, and the other is to use alternatives to food.

By snacking on healthful foods consistently, you can control appetite, avoid becoming anxious about hunger, and avoid building up a need for a binge to provide pleasure. Food has the greatest effects on pleasure responses when you have not eaten for a while. If you starve yourself and then binge, the intense relief of bingeing will be positive reinforcement to do it again. If you eat moderately and consistently, you avoid this strong emotional influence.

You can also use alternatives to eating for pleasure. Physical activity is very important to mental health, and by relieving anxiety or tension, can actually reduce the desire to eat. One of the well-known effects of physical activity is the release of pleasure-promoting chemicals called endorphins. These chemicals are the mediators of the famous "runner's high." Much of the pleasure response provided by fat and sugar is also caused by endorphins, so physical activity makes a nearly ideal alternative, and one that confers health benefits of its own. Other pleasurable activities, such as a soothing bath or listening to music, or dancing to your favorite tunes, may also work for you as food substitutes; these, too, can trigger an endorphin release.

Combining a realistic view of pleasure from food with a healthful dietary pattern is powerful. The one will help you realize that choosing foods based on health can increase your pleasure. And the other will cause you to get more pleasure from the very foods that promote your health. Recall that familiarity is an important determinant of our dietary preferences, and eating what we prefer influences pleasure. So, by getting used to a healthful diet, you make that diet more pleasurable.

Don't Put Up with Neurochemical Nonsense!

There is good evidence that the more fat we eat, the more we tend to like fat. The same seems to be true of sugar and salt. All of these responses are driven by chemicals released when we eat, or produced from the foods we eat. Weaving together various lines of evidence in the medical literature, an important pattern emerges. It appears that this so-called "neurochemistry" of eating is very important, because it sets in motion desires and cravings not under your control.

What you can control, however, is the dietary pattern that sets these chemical reactions in motion in the first place. In general, eating a healthful diet helps to coordinate and discipline your neurochemical reactions; eating a highly processed, unbalanced diet does just the opposite. While making a change to more healthful eating is challenging just because it is change, eating well tends to reinforce itself in many ways, including brain chemistry.

When Food Talks, Listen

Finally, pay attention to your needs for food as a source of pleasure. They tell you something about yourself. If you are eating in an unrestrained way, or bingeing, you may be using food to fill a need for something else. Perhaps you are working too hard, or not getting enough recreation. You may be bored, stressed, or unhappy. These are important issues in your life, and should not be buried under chips or cheese or candy bars. Be honest with yourself about what you are eating, and why, and your diet may well lead you to other important ways of improving your health, both physical and emotional.

Obstacle/Opportunity 4: Food as Self-punishment

Food is what we often turn to when we need comfort. But, because food, or what we do with it, is involved in weight gain and obesity, the very thing we turn to for feeling good can also make us feel bad. And if you start feeling badly about your interactions with food and the effects they have on you, you may start using food to punish yourself. Many people "atone" for an occasional indulgence by indulging even more. That leads to feeling really badly, which is the punishment. But none of this is useful, or even reasonable. Gaining a good understanding of this dangerous cycle can take it out of your way, and give you one less obstacle to worry about.

Strategy

The first goal here is to appreciate that there is never a reason to punish yourself for the way you eat. Never!

Either you are eating the way you want to, or not. If not, there is a reason. It may be an emotional need, or hunger, or tension.

But, as you well know, if you overeat often, or eat the "wrong" foods in the wrong amounts, you will pay a price. So while you should not punish yourself for indulging, you do want to defend against it.

Live & Let Lapse

Many of the skills and strategies you've gained along the *way to eat* will help you avoid the situations that will tempt you to punish yourself with food.

The more you get used to good dietary habits, the less susceptible you become to bingeing. But no matter how good your skills, and how sophisticated your strategies, you will still be human! You might slip. Do for yourself what you would probably do for anyone else—give a hand up, not a swift kick. Satisfy your occasional craving, indulge an intermittent need to splurge, and move on. Nutritional health and weight control are not the product of what you eat today, or ate yesterday; they are the product of your usual way of eating every day. If you are moving toward a healthful pattern of eating, an occasional lapse is not harmful.

In fact, it can even be helpful. Whatever your skills and strategies, a lapse suggests there may be a hole in your defenses against the nutritional environment. Take a look at it. Be interested, not upset, or disappointed in yourself, or angry. What obstacle got in your way and caused you to stumble? You are increasingly an expert in following the healthful *way to eat*, so running into an occasional obstacle will not stop your progress. Every lapse is a lesson. You now have one more strategy, one more defense.

Little by little, as you add the lessons each lapse teaches to your growing array of skills and strategies, you will simply stop having lapses. Until then, see them as part of the process. You don't need to be perfect to be really good!

Obstacle/Opportunity 5: Night-eating Disorder

For the most part, this book does not address any actual eating disorders. But we are all subject to some degree of "disordered" eating. Some eating disorders share so much with "normal" disordered eating that they warrant discussion as obstacles to eating well. Even so, if you have any concerns about a possible eating disorder in yourself or a loved one, please do not use this, or any book, as a substitute for medical attention and advice.

The night-eating syndrome consists of sleeplessness (insomnia), hunger and eating at night, and a relative lack of appetite first thing in the morning. While the actual disorder may not be all that common, features of it are. You don't need to have a disorder to have a tendency to skip breakfast, and to be hungry in the evening and at night.

This pattern can of course lead to weight gain, as well as impaired sleep. There is a neurochemical basis for the condition, meaning that chemical messengers to the brain are responsible, or at least involved. In particular, levels of *melatonin*, a hormone produced by the pineal gland, tend not to rise at night as they should. Levels of *leptin*, a hormone influencing appetite, also tend to be low, while levels of the stress hormone *cortisol* tend to be high. The various features of this syndrome, whether or not they are part of any true disorder, can often be managed effectively by eating well.

Strategy

Many of the strategies already provided for controlling appetite and hunger are a defense against night-eating as well. Place an emphasis on complex carbohydrates in your diet from whole grains, beans, and legumes. Such foods, along with fruits and vegetables, provide an abundance of fiber. Soluble fiber in particular is beneficial in providing slow, steady entry of glucose and fat molecules into the bloodstream. This, in turn, keeps insulin levels moderate. This pattern is helpful in preventing sudden spikes in hunger. By eating complex carbohydrates consistently, serotonin and melatonin levels can be boosted, improving both mood and sleep.

Eating relatively small meals, or snacks, regularly throughout the day can be helpful as well. Less insulin is needed when foods are spread out. Less insulin generally means less hunger, and higher levels of leptin. This can help prevent a surge in appetite in the evening.

While eating breakfast at a particular time is not necessary, avoiding long periods without eating is. An overnight fast is already many hours without eating, so breakfast can be quite important. Eating a small amount in the morning may help to achieve the small, frequent spacing of meals or snacks throughout the day that can be used to prevent hunger at night.

Stuffing Your Way to Being Hungry

Avoid having a large meal late in the day, which can trigger a strong insulin response. This, in turn, rushes glucose into cells, and may actually push glucose levels to, or past, the lower limits of normal. This results in *hypoglycemia*, or low blood sugar, which leads in turn to more hunger. Odd as it may seem, a big dinner may lead to, rather than prevent, more hunger, and eating, during the night.

A large meal late in the day can be avoided by eating small amounts throughout the day. Consider a late afternoon snack consisting of fresh or dried fruit, nonfat yogurt or whole-grain products, or fresh vegetables such as baby carrots, specifically as a means of reducing and controlling your appetite before dinner.

If you do get hungry at night, decide in advance what foods are acceptable. By eating nutritious, fiber-rich foods, such as dried fruit, you can start to gain mastery over the features of the night-eating disorder even when you need to give in to them. On any given day, eat only one food if you eat at night. This will help avoid the hazards of sensory specific satiety, and limit the calories you take in.

Have a Good Night

Finally, assess the quality of your sleep, and the reasons why it might not be too good. Are you anxious or stressed? Do you have any time to relax before going to bed? If you sleep soundly, you won't be up looking for something to eat! Try to find some relaxing routine that helps you transition from the demands of the day to restful sleep. If insomnia is a serious problem for you, consult a health-care professional.

Obstacle/Opportunity 6: Nutrition Nostalgia

Our memories have a powerful influence on our emotions. And this may be especially true when it comes to food and flavors. Much of our sense of taste is actually smell, and the nerve cells we use for our sense of smell run directly into very primitive parts of our brain. So, reactions in this system can affect us to the very core.

Because of this, we are all strongly influenced by our food memories. The smell of freshly baked bread, a backyard barbecue, Christmas or Thanksgiving dinner—these aromas, and the memories to which they are linked, exert a strong influence on our dietary preferences. If you grew up eating a healthful diet, this force will help keep you eating well. But if your food memories are matched to a diet high in fat, or sugar, or salt, this powerful, emotional drive may be trying to tug you from your new way of eating, back to the old.

Strategy

Begin to address and overcome food nostalgia by making slow adjustments to your diet, and by preserving foods and dishes that matter most to you. Little by little, you can modify even your favorite dishes by using newly acquired knowledge of ingredient substitutions, recipes, and cooking techniques or by sharing this information with whomever does the cooking in your home.

When you do this, you maintain the appearance of much of your diet, along with its familiar flavors and aromas. This way, you use nostalgia to your advantage, tapping into a long-standing preference for dishes that now fit in well with a healthful way of eating. But if your favorite dish just does not taste the same with healthy substitutions that's ok also. You can still eat it in moderation.

Only Follow Your Nose if It Leads the Right Way!

Just as knowledge about how to eat well must be used to protect against some of the misleading messages conveyed by pleasure from eating, this knowledge must be used to deal with nostalgia. You may have strong memories and nostalgia for the bacon you ate at breakfast every morning growing up. You now know, however, that eating bacon each morning for breakfast is not nearly the best you can do nutritionally. Identify the ways in which nostalgia is working against you, and exert particular effort there.

On the other hand, don't resist nostalgia's lure too intensely. You may have strong food memories associated, for example, with holidays or special occasions. If you eat well most of the time, you can certainly indulge in an old favorite several times a year, no matter what its nutritional composition!

Finally, don't overlook the ways in which you can use food nostalgia to help others, specifically, your children. You can be the reason that your kids associate good times, fun, family, and comfort with foods and a diet that promote their health.

Obstacle/Opportunity 7: Premenstrual Syndrome

Premenstrual syndrome (PMS) is clearly related to the hormonal variations of the menstrual cycle, but why some women get it and some do not cannot yet be determined.

Appetite, hunger, satiety (fullness), cravings, and aversions all vary with the menstrual cycle. These variations are subtle in many women, but quite profound in others. In the most extreme manifestation, the premenstrual syndrome is associated with very strong food preferences that are thought to represent an attempt at self-treatment. The opposite is also true; dietary pattern, and body weight, may influence susceptibility to PMS. Variation in eating pattern and appetite is a well-recognized occurrence in even normal menstrual cycles.

PMS is very common in the U.S. Severe symptoms occur in up to 10 percent of all susceptible women, while up to 40 percent experience less severe symptoms. Premenstrual symptoms consistent with the syndrome occur in up to 60 percent of women!

There are four distinct symptom patterns: anxiety is prominent in one, depression in another, food cravings in another, and bloating (hyperhydration) in the last. Treatment may work best when matched to the specific symptom pattern, but there is a role for dietary and nutrient interventions in all four variants.

If you have PMS, you may need to seek medical attention for it, along with applying the dietary recommendations offered here.

Strategy

Even if PMS results in cravings, and binges, this need not upset your overall dietary pattern. After all, these symptoms come along only for a few days each month.

So, an important strategy for preventing PMS-related damage to your diet is to eat well in general. Of course, you should not punish yourself if PMS does lead to a binge. Accept it, and move on.

Also, don't fight cravings when they occur, but do manage them. Eat the food or type of food your craving is calling for (chocolate is a common choice) rather than trying to avoid it. But practice some portion control, so that even a splurge does not involve a great excess of calories.

The same dietary pattern that will prevent PMS from harming your overall nutritional health may help prevent or control PMS as well. Such a diet is rich in vitamins, minerals, and other micronutrients, helps to control weight, and helps to produce and maintain adequate levels of brain chemicals such as serotonin. All of these effects have the potential to reduce the symptoms of PMS.

In addition, nutritional supplements that show promise in managing PMS, including calcium, magnesium, essential fatty acids, and to a lesser extent vitamin B6, are often reasonable additions to the diet just for purposes of health promotion. And the other strategies that may help control the syndrome—limiting caffeine intake, avoiding nicotine, and being physically active—are all indicated for health promotion as well. So, by taking care of PMS, you wind up taking good care of your overall health, and vice versa.

Serotonin, Again

Serotonin levels are thought to be related to symptoms of PMS, accounting for the carbohydrate craving experienced by some women. Consistent with this theory is evidence that drugs that raise serotonin, such as Prozac, relieve symptoms in many women, especially those with the depressive variant of the syndrome. Eating a diet rich in complex carbohydrate and fiber can help keep serotonin levels stable at an adequate level, and may provide some of the same benefits as these antidepressant medications.

Finally, while there is considerable interest in plant estrogens (called *phytoestrogens*) in managing PMS, their effects are not yet known. Nonetheless, incorporating soy into the diet is advisable on general principles, as soy provides excellent protein, essential fatty acids, and a range of nutrients along with its phytoestrogens.

Obstacle/Opportunity 8: Seasonal Affective Disorder

Seasonal affective disorder is a condition of sadness, or depression, that occurs during the winter months. The condition is relatively common where winters are long and harsh and daylight hours are limited; it does not occur in the tropics. As a result, there is reason to believe that sunlight is a factor. Sunlight influences production of the brain hormone melatonin, and leads to the production of vitamin D, also a hormone, in the skin. When sun exposure is limited, levels of melatonin, vitamin D, and serotonin tend to be low. All of these reactions may contribute to the syndrome, abbreviated SAD, although the actual cause is uncertain.

Because serotonin levels tend to be low in SAD, there is an urge to eat carbohydrate; as discussed, carbohydrates can boost serotonin levels. However, in the modern diet, the carbohydrate people tend to reach for comes from highly processed foods, often full of sugar, fat, and calories, and relatively low in fiber and nutrients. These foods naturally contribute to weight gain. And, since this craving for carbohydrate comes along in winter when physical activity levels tend to be lower, a formula for seasonal weight gain is created. Thus, SAD, and attempts to self-treat with processed carbohydrate, can represent an obstacle to healthful eating year round.

The syndrome of SAD can often be controlled by eating well. But, it can also require medical attention. Recommendations are provided here for a dietary pattern that will help prevent and control symptoms of SAD. These recommendations should be in addition to, but not instead of, any professional medical advice you or a loved one may need to treat the disorder effectively.

Strategy

Remember that not all carbohydrate is created equal. Processed carbohydrate—chips, snack foods, packaged desserts—often comes along with added sugar, fat, and salt, and very limited fiber. While these foods may temporarily boost serotonin levels, and improve mood, the effect will quickly fade.

Foods rich in complex carbohydrate, including whole-grain breads, whole-grain cereals, cooked grains, beans, lentils, seeds, fruits, and vegetables are the very foods upon which a healthful dietary pattern is based. These foods provide the kind of carbohydrate that will support serotonin levels without leading to weight gain, and without promoting cycles of "surges" and "crashes" in mood. Complex carbohydrate has staying power.

In combination with a health-promoting dietary pattern, sun exposure is helpful. Weather and circumstances permitting, bundle up and try to make the outdoors part of your life, even in winter. If ambitious, consider skiing, skating, snowboarding, or snowshoeing. If less ambitious, get similar benefits from going for a walk, or sledding. The combination of sunlight exposure, and good physical activity, is particularly beneficial to mood, health, and weight control.

Other than lifestyle, supplements or medication might be useful. A daily supplement of vitamin D is most promising thus far. If SAD is severe, you should consult a health care professional; treatment with an antidepressant that raises serotonin levels is sometimes appropriate.

You Can Try Some Things at Home…But Not This
Finally, you might consider moving to Hawaii! This works every time, or so we hear.

Obstacle/Opportunity 9: Stress

Stress, and related conditions, such as tension, anxiety, frustration, or sadness, can influence all of our behaviors. Because eating is one of the more controllable and available sources of pleasure and comfort, it is quite natural to use food to alleviate stress.

But if you eat when you are hungry, then eat some more when you are stressed, and perhaps eat some more when sad, or celebrating, or bored, it adds up to too much eating!

The Then/Now Conflict

The basic stress response is well understood. Traditionally referred to as the "flight or fight" response, it describes the release of hormones called catecholamines—especially epinephrine (adrenaline) and norepineph-rine (noradrenaline)—and the physical responses to this hormone surge. Those responses include increased heart rate and blood pressure, dilated pupils, dilated breathing passages, and a surge of blood into muscles. This reaction prepares us to fight or flee, and it served our ancestors well.

It serves us less well. At work, giving a talk, teaching, paying taxes, or doing any of the many things we all need to do in our lives, there is very little opportunity to run away, or fight! In fact, these are almost never the right response. So, we're left with flight-or-fight hormones, and we just accumulate the stress! And as we do, we turn to our old standby— food—to help us out of our troubles.

Strategy

Take stock of stress in your life. Consider the things you do that cause you to feel tense or anxious. Try to make changes that reduce your stress level. Consider a course in stress management. A certified stress-management counselor can teach you to control the flight or fight response so you are not filled to the brim with hormones you can't use as nature intended. Your medical provider should be able to help you find a stress management counselor, or you might try the yellow pages, a local spa, or an area gym. Stress management can take many forms, from breathing exercises, to yoga, to meditation.

Avoid letting stress build up during the day. If possible, try to work out some of your tension in physical activity, which is exactly what the primitive stress response is designed for. Use food to help handle stress, but use it wisely. Chewing can be a way to work out tension; many of us clench our jaws or grind our teeth when stressed. As previously discussed, snacking regularly confers many benefits if the snacks are well chosen; it can be useful for controlling stress, as well. Throughout the day, have dried fruit or whole-grain breads or cereals handy. All of these foods are substantial, and satisfying to chew. In addition to controlling appetite and providing good nutrition, these foods help relieve stress directly. They offer the additional benefit of increasing serotonin levels, which helps to restore a sense of calm. Avoid going for long periods without eating; doing so can add to your stress level.

By combining several simple strategies, you can use your way of eating to manage stress, rather than being stressed into eating badly.

Step 6:

Negotiate the Modern Nutritional Environment

THE MODERN ENVIRONMENT offers some clear advantages to us. We can all be thankful for the benefits of shelter, heat, sanitation, and so forth. Our life expectancy increased nearly thirty-five years in the twentieth century, due mostly to improvements in the environment. But be that as it may, the modern environment, nutritional and otherwise, is significantly at odds with our Stone Age adaptations.

Technology and convenience devices make it possible to avoid physical activity, while demanding work schedules make it difficult to find the time to compensate with exercise. Nutrient-dilute, calorie-dense, tasty, and tempting food abounds, and is accessible to most of us, most of the time. Added to the challenges of a fast-food, drive-through, remote-control culture is the confusion generated by a barrage of misleading messages in food advertisements and on food product labels.

Thus, the modern environment represents a fundamental and formidable challenge to nutritional health. As with so many of the other potential barriers to nutritional health, converting obstacles to opportunity begins quite simply by recognizing they are there:

1) *Building Design*
2) *Convenience Devices*
3) *Convenient Availability of Non-nutritious Foods*
4) *Fast-food Restaurant Proliferation*

    5) Flavor Manipulation

    6) Food Advertising Directed at Children

    7) Food Label Pitfalls

    8) Food Supply Globalization

    9) Inconvenience Involved in Finding, Ordering, or Preparing Nutritious Foods

    10) Internet Use & Video Games

    11) Misleading Menus

    12) School Practices

    13) Sedentary Pastimes

    14) Suburban Design Issues

    15) Weight Loss Industry Claims/Unregulated Products

Each aspect of the modern environment that is understood as a potential threat to eating well and being physically activity is one less aspect of the environment you will ignore, take for granted, or simply accept. The more obstacles you recognize, the more opportunities you create. And as with the other categories of obstacles, the conversion of these to opportunities benefits from a certain "economy of scale." Impediments to eating well, and being physically active, are interrelated—and so are the strategies for overcoming them.

Thus, each skill, each strategy—even if directed at only a single obstacle—is likely to convert several others into opportunities for better health as well. Most of what you need to know, and to do, to navigate safely through the modern nutritional environment is based on skills and strategies you have picked up by now.

Obstacle/Opportunity 1: Building Design

Think about any large building you've ever visited (and perhaps even one you work in every day). As you enter the lobby, which is easier to find, the stairs, or the elevator? And if you do happen to check out both, which has wood paneling, and which concrete walls? Which is well lit and plays music?

Even in the ways we design our buildings, we prioritize convenience over health needs. The stairs represent an opportunity for physical activity that a whole array of cues, both blatant and subtle, prompt us

---

Only in the Funny Papers, Right?...

Newspaper cartoon: a group of women are standing next to a stairwell wearing gym clothes. The sign above the stairs says, *"Aerobics Class, 2nd Floor."* They are waiting for the elevator...

---

to avoid. This, along with countless other influences that reduce our physical activity, make us more susceptible to weight gain even if our food energy intake is moderate.

Strategy

The first thing to do when confronting the options afforded by the modern environment, including the use of elevators and escalators, is to remember they are *options*, not obligations. We have established the use of elevators rather than stairs as the cultural norm to such an extent that use of stairs may feel strange, or "abnormal." But if so, we have let technology run away with us! Instead of replacing the obligation of physical work with options, we have replaced it with the obligation to be sedentary! Technology is supposed to serve us, not the other way around!

So, if your health and joints permit (and most do), use the stairs instead of the elevator or escalator. To be reasonable about it, set some appropriate limits. For example, use the stairs for any trip between the first and fourth floors; use of the elevator for higher floors is not unreasonable. As your fitness improves, you may want to gradually move up your threshold, to the fifth, or even sixth floor.

Be aware of the seductive power of cultural norms, and be prepared to resist them when they don't make sense. We bypass opportunities for physical activity all of the time, even as some of us go out of our way to reintroduce some physical activity into our mostly sedentary lives.

All physical activity counts. *Healthy People 2010* uses thirty minutes of accumulated, moderate physical activity on most days of the week as a goal for the U.S. population. Each use of the stairs contributes to that total, as does every other thing you do during the day that is kinetic, or "in motion."

Of course, the ultimate goal for us all as we confront and surmount health barriers in the modern environment should be to remove the barriers altogether. So, for example, stairs should be easy to find, paneled, well-lit, and filled with music (perhaps at some time in the future, there will be no "elevator music," but "stair music" instead!). Elevators should be a little harder to find, or available only to those with handicaps, and/or available only to the fourth floor and higher. When the environment encourages rather than discourages physical activity, it becomes much easier to be physically active.

Obstacle/Opportunity 2: Convenience Devices

The development of each new convenience device tends to eliminate one more source of physical activity from a typical day. From cars to dishwashers, ride-on lawn mowers to food processors, escalators to remote controls, drive-through restaurants to snowblowers, our environment is cluttered with the many products of our resourcefulness that make it easier and easier for us to avoid physical activity altogether.

The Then/Now Conflict

Most creatures are physically active when, and because, they have to be, not by choice. In fact, nature tends to be conservative about energy expenditure, because burning calories you may not be able to replace is not conducive to survival. Our ancestors were not physical activity enthusiasts, and certainly didn't need to be. They just did what they had to do to survive. And doing so meant enormous physical activity.

As a result, we are well adapted to a high level of physical activity. One aspect of that adaptation is metabolic efficiency, the ability to run for a long time on relatively few calories. Another is that the less we do, the lower our basal metabolism, enabling us to become even more metabolically efficient when inactive.

While physical activity levels have gradually declined over much of the historical era, the period since the Industrial Revolution, and especially over the latter half of the twentieth century, has seen much more accelerated declines. As technology gives rise to ever more technology, we are completely remaking the environment in which we live. Already, physical activity is almost completely avoidable. For the first time in all of human history, therefore, you have to try to be physically active, rather than be physically active to survive.

Physical activity and nutrition really cannot be considered separately from one another. Both relate to energy balance, and therefore weight. Both also make vital contributions to insulin levels, glycogen and fat storage, and protein metabolism. The evidence is clear that physical activity is essential for our Stone Age bodies to be in good health, and to maintain weight, or weight loss, over time.

Strategy

There is, basically, just one way to avoid the reduction, or elimination, of physical activity in your daily routine as a result of energy-saving devices: don't use them! Or, more precisely, don't use them all, all of the time.

Clearly, it is very difficult, if not impossible, to give up all, or even most, of the technology that is a part of everyday life. But if you recognize that each use of technology in place of your muscles is a threat to your health, you can make some informed choices.

Hand-washing a few dishes, and using the dishwasher only for larger loads, may not sound like fun, but it can burn some calories, and help the environment in the bargain. Using a leaf blower in flowerbeds, but then resorting to the time-honored rake out on the lawn can turn yard work into an excellent aerobic activity. Sweeping confers a similar benefit. Climbing stairs, opening a garage door, getting up to change a channel, and pushing a lawn mower all could contribute to the physical activity in your typical day, or week, or year.

Use Technology, Selectively

As you look for ways to build physical activity back into your life, don't be too demanding of yourself. For example, while standing up to change the television channel is "better" than use of a remote control in terms of physical activity, it can be pretty tedious if you have several hundred channels! In that case, decide that this is a convenience device worth using. But don't give in, unthinkingly, to use of them all.

Decide which conveniences you value the most, and make use of those. In other instances, you can perhaps decide that the benefit of some physical activity exceeds the benefit of convenience, and take a more old-fashioned approach.

Above all, be aware. Assess your activity level as you go through a typical day or week. Consider all of the times you avoid physical exertion by use of technology. Attentiveness to the many ways technology sneaks into our lives to reduce our physical activity enables you to blend the best of convenience and health.

Obstacle/Opportunity 4
Fast-food Restaurant Proliferation

In general, fast food is energy dense (often fried), relatively nutrient-poor, low in fiber, high in salt and fat and sugar, very tasty, inexpensive, and, of course, fast, therefore convenient. For busy people, this combination, along with a drive-through window, is an almost irresistible temptation. Add to this the proliferation of fast-food franchises, so that everywhere you go you pass one, or several, and a well-financed advertising campaign, and you have a very clear and present threat to our best nutritional intentions!

Strategy

Begin with a simple, clear truth: a poor diet will threaten your health, and undermine your efforts to control your weight. You must compare these costs to the benefits of fast food—its convenience, taste, price— and make a decision. What are your priorities? Chances are, you want it all. You would like to have convenience, taste, value, along with good health and weight control. Right? Let's see how close we can get.

Make New Food Friends, but Keep (Some of) the Old
Any food, no matter how high in fat, or salt, or sugar or calories, can be consistent with good eating habits if consumed in appropriate moderation, in the context of a healthful dietary pattern. So, if you or your family particularly like certain fast foods, they can remain a part of your diet—as long as they are not the major part of your diet.

Button Up Your Overcoat…And Zip Up Your Lunch Bag
Because the spread of fast-food restaurants makes it likely you will encounter them often, one of the key defenses is to plan your daily diet

---

Of CABG's & Kings...

You know the names of the popular fast-food restaurants; there is no need to mention them. But CABG? That stands for "coronary artery bypass graft"—the surgery done when the blood vessels that supply the heart are all gummed up. High-fat fast food contributes to high cholesterol levels; high cholesterol is a leading risk factor for coronary artery disease; and coronary artery disease is what makes CABG necessary.

So...be careful what way you have it, and what arches you pass under. Or you may be headed through the looking glass...and toward the operating room!

---

in advance. Just as you would be subject to dehydration if you wandered into the desert without water, or frostbite if you wandered onto the tundra without boots and gloves, you are subject to the hazards of the modern nutritional environment unless you anticipate them, and plan accordingly.

Fast food is an excellent example. If you find yourself "out there," hungry, without food available, and no prior planning, what are you likely to encounter? Fast food. And if you don't have another option, fast food is what you will eat.

So you must have another option almost all of the time if you want to approach a good way of eating. Have nutritious snacks or meals readily available when you leave home, and commit in advance to eating what you have prepared. Decide beforehand, not when tempted, which restaurants or food choices are acceptable, and which are not, for any given meal, or day.

Eating fast food every day simply because fast-food restaurants are everywhere is allowing yourself to be manipulated, and your health and that of your family to be compromised. Take charge, make the rules, and set appropriate limits for fast food in your life.

Obstacle/Opportunity 5: Flavor Manipulation

We tend to eat more when we have access to a wider variety of flavors due to the taste thresholds in the satiety center of our brain. This would be enough of a challenge if we were in charge of the variety in our diets, but often, we are not.

Modern food processing introduces variety that goes well beyond what occurs in nature, modifying food from its natural state for a variety of purposes, among them to improve taste and palatability, to stimulate appetite, to improve safety, to extend shelf life, to enhance presentation, or to improve convenience. Some of these practices are at times neutral or even beneficial in terms of health, but many are not.

Processed foods often have long ingredient lists that include various flavor enhancers, often in unexpected categories. For example, breakfast cereals and desserts may contain considerable amounts of salt, and salty or snack foods may contain considerable sugar, as shown in the ingredient lists for A) General Mills Cheerios breakfast cereal, and B) Heinz Tomato Ketchup. Cheerios provide 280 mg of sodium per 110 kcal serving. All of the 23 kcal per Tbsp. serving of Heinz ketchup come from sugar.

A) Cheerios Ingredient List:

> WHOLE-GRAIN OATS (INCLUDE OAT BRAN), MODIFIED CORN STARCH, WHEAT STARCH, SUGAR, SALT, CALCIUM CARBONATE, OAT FIBER, TRISODIUM PHOSPHATE, VITAMIN E (MIXED TOCOPHEROLS) ADDED TO PRESERVE FRESHNESS

B) Heinz Tomato Ketchup Ingredient List:

> TOMATO CONCENTRATE MADE FROM RED RIPE TOMATOES, DISTILLED VINEGAR, HIGH FRUCTOSE CORN SYRUP, CORN SYRUP, SALT, SPICE, ONION POWDER, NATURAL FLAVORING

The only way for your overall diet (of 2,000 calories per day) to have the recommended 2,400 mg per day of sodium or less is for the average sodium content of the foods you eat to be less than 1.2 mg per calorie. In the case of Cheerios, there are 2.5 mg of sodium per calorie! This means that your breakfast cereal may be more than twice as salty as your overall diet should be! If you have that much sodium in your diet before ever getting to the snack foods you know are salty, what hope is there of meeting the guidelines?

Of course, your breakfast cereal does not need to put you over the salt threshold. For example, New Morning Brand Oatios, a relatively unprocessed product otherwise much like Cheerios, provides just 10 mg of sodium per 120 kcal serving, or less than 0.1 mg of sodium per calorie!

Similarly, dietary recommendations call for limiting simple sugars to less than 10 percent of total calories. In the case of the ketchup, 100 percent of the calories come from sugar. So just as you are adding salt to your diet before finishing breakfast, you are also adding sugar before ever getting to dessert! And foods not expected to contain added fat, such as bread or granola, often do contain added fat.

The above examples help to make an important point: expect the unexpected when it comes to the ingredients in processed foods. Just be aware of how even some of the foods you turn to for good nutrition might contribute to an excess of sugar, salt, or fat.

Strategy

To prevent undue influence on your eating of flavor enhancers in processed foods, the first, best step is to limit your intake of processed foods. This occurs on its own if you base your diet mostly on grains, fruits, vegetables, and other natural foods. This is the same pattern that is recommended for health promotion and weight control: how convenient!

Boxes, Bottles, & Bags: Oh, My!

Whenever eating foods in cans, jars, bags, or boxes, take a look at the ingredient and nutrition labels (guidance for doing so is provided in Section IV). Look for sodium in sweet or breakfast foods, added sugar in salty or snack foods, or added oil/fat. Keep in mind that many of these ingredients influence appetite, even though you may not taste them when you eat the product.

Less Is More, or at Least Better

In most categories of processed food, from canned tuna to breakfast cereal, crackers to ketchup, bread to baked beans, there are choices with more or less added flavor enhancers. In general, the options with less added salt, sugar, oil, and/or chemical additives are preferred. In each category, getting to know the specific products, or brands, that avoid excess additives will help you avoid the risk of too many flavor temptations, as well as unnecessary additions of fat and calories. Recommended foods and product lines are provided in Section IV.

Tolerate Transition Time

Making any change in your diet is challenging at first. If you do try to convert to new brands or products, commit roughly two weeks to the transition. If you stick with the new product for one to two weeks, it will taste appropriate, and the old choice won't taste as good.

Obstacle/Opportunity 6
Food Advertising Directed at Children

One of the challenges for any adult attempting to eat well is the need to satisfy the dietary preferences of others in the household, especially children. And among the factors shaping the dietary preferences of children is advertising that makes sugary and salty snacks irresistibly appealing.

During the course of a typical year, the average child between the ages of two and seven in the U.S. spends roughly 2.5 hours per day watching television. During each hour of television, there are approximately twenty commercials, and about half of these, on average, are for food items. As a result, the preschool to kindergarten age child in the U.S. sees some 9,125 food commercials during the course of a typical year! Roughly two billion dollars are spent in the U.S. each year on food promotion, and some seven billion dollars on television advertising. More than 50 percent of TV ads for foods are devoted to convenience/fast foods, snacks, alcohol, and soft drinks. Only 2 percent of all food advertising is for fruits, vegetables, and grains combined! The National Cancer Institute's five-a-day program spends one million dollars per year, less than one dollar for every three thousand dollars the food industry spends on television ads for junk food! The appeal of advertised foods to children is enhanced by linking them to popular television or movie characters. The inclusion of popular "action figures" in fast-food meals or packaged food items makes these items even more appealing to children, and that much harder for parents to resist.

Dietitian Chronicles...

Doug and Amy were concerned about their daughter, Emily. At age eight, she was already clearly overweight. So they came in, seeking advice.

Did they encourage her to clean her plate? *Eh...yes.*

Did they use dessert as a reward if she *did* clean her plate? *Ummm...yes.*

Did she ask for foods she saw advertised on television? *Of course.*

Did they buy those foods for her? *Well...how could you resist?*

We'll leave the rest of the discussion to your imagination!

Strategy

The first step in combating the influence of food advertisement on your children is to recognize that there is such an influence, and that it may be quite strong. Children are literally bombarded with food advertisements while watching television, and will want to eat what they see advertised. You must therefore be prepared to contend with this want.

There are some things your kids see on television that you may be willing for them to have. There are others you are not. Wherever you draw the line, *do* draw the line somewhere, letting your kids know they can't always get what they want!

But to do this with food requires overcoming a potential barrier having much more to do with parents than children. If you are like most parents, you actually want your children to have preferred foods, so that they will eat. Most young children are somewhat fussy. Parents are thus often contending with the challenge of talking their children *into* eating.

Enough Is Enough

But it is time, indeed past time, for parents in the industrialized world to revisit the tendency to encourage their children to eat more. There is evidence, going back nearly a century, that simply when provided access to a variety of nutritious foods, young children make choices that meet all of their nutritional needs. This nutrient balance may not be achieved every day, and certainly not every meal, but will occur over the span of every few days. Thus, as a parent you need to be secure in the knowledge that your children, given access to an adequate diet, will not starve themselves!

Quality, Not Quantity
So, the second step in combating the influence of media ads on the food preferences of your children is to care more about the quality of your children's nutrition, than its quantity. This sounds obvious once stated, but is not, in our combined thirty-five years of nutrition counseling experience, characteristic of most parents' behavior. You can accomplish a good deal by making it characteristic of yours.

Tacos…and the Terminator
There is much concern about the effects of media violence on children's behavior, and three principal suggestions from experts to limit the damage. *First*, television violence should be reduced and/or regulated so that children are not excessively or inappropriately exposed. *Second*, parents should monitor and control the television viewing of their own children to limit adverse exposures. And *third*, to the extent that children will see violence on television, parents should interpret it for their children, so that reality and fantasy, the appropriate versus the inappropriate, are understood.

All three of these recommendations apply just as well to food advertising. There is interest among experts in regulating food advertising to children. In the meantime, parents should factor this exposure in to their decisions about their children's TV viewing. Know that if you let your child watch several hours of television, they will likely see dozens of advertisements for sugary, high-calorie, high-fat, relatively non-nutritious food products. But, it may be unrealistic for you to prevent your children from having this exposure, in which case, you are left with the third and final recommendation: help your kids to understand it.

Of Diet & Danger
We routinely talk to our children about age-appropriate dangers in the environment: talking to strangers, bullies, cigarettes, drugs, alcohol, and

sex. In a society so prone to adverse health effects of dietary excesses, food needs to be added to the list.

Recognize that dietary preferences established in childhood are strong determinants of later preferences. Many risk factors for chronic disease, including those related to diet, have their origins in childhood. Consider your family history. Is there cancer, or heart disease, or diabetes in the family? If so, your children may be at higher than average risk for these conditions. Their lifestyle and eating habits can either aggravate that risk, or provide excellent defense against it. You are addressing your responsibilities as a parent far better by guiding your children toward healthful eating than you are by simply encouraging them to eat, or letting them eat whatever they want.

Finally, your own diet will exert a strong influence on the impressions and preferences of your children. Your religion, your holidays, your clothes, and your traditions may differ from what your children see on television, but they come to learn that this is the way it is in *their* family. So, too, with eating.

Make healthful eating a family tradition. That way, your children help reinforce your commitment to dietary health, even as you help establish a pattern that will promote their health throughout life.

Obstacle/Opportunity 7: Food Label Pitfalls

Food labels are supposed to provide information that helps us make choices about what to eat. But food package information can be manipulated to convey messages that enhance the attractiveness of a food product. For example, when the health benefits of oat bran were first being popularized, a vast array of food products listed "oat bran" in bold letters on their packages, no matter how trivial an amount they actually contained. In some cases, a wand dipped in oat bran may have been ever-so-gently waved over the vat!

Among the labeling practices in wide use are "contains no cholesterol," "lite," "fat-free," and "all natural." Each of these, and many others, address some of the current, popular concerns about nutrition. Many of these claims, however, are misleading, if not deceptive. In buying food, as in all buying, the adage *caveat emptor*, or "buyer beware," is appropriate.

Modern Oils...A Tragi-Comedy in Three Parts...

1) The food industry previously used animal fat, such as lard, as a pre-ferred fat in processed foods. When enough consumers learned about the adverse health effects of this practice, and voiced their opinion by the way they shopped, the food industry moved on...

2) ...to tropical vegetable oils, including palm oil, palm kernel oil, and coconut oil, which sounded better than lard, but have the same health effects! So the industry again move on...

3) ...to partially hydrogenated oils, which are just as bad!

What happens next? I guess it's up to us...and them!

Strategy

The motto of the Sym's clothing store is "an educated consumer is our best customer." This is certainly true with regard to food purchasing. The potential obstacle of misleading food packages is converted into an opportunity for prudent food purchases if you become an "educated consumer."

There are three steps involved in becoming an educated food consumer. First, adopt the *caveat emptor* ("buyer beware") philosophy—beware of misleading sales pitches, and select foods you know will promote your well-being. Second, you must know what makes up a healthful eating pattern, which you have been learning throughout this book. And finally, you must know how to interpret food packages, ingredient lists, and nutrition labels. The claims made on food packages are regulated by the United States Food and Drug Administration (FDA) in the case of processed foods, or the United States Department of Agriculture (USDA) in the case of agricultural products. But there is considerable leeway in the regulations. For example, it is perfectly acceptable, and indeed accurate, to note on a bottle of corn oil that it "contains no cholesterol." The information, however, is of no actual value. Cholesterol is an animal product—no vegetable oil contains any cholesterol! So, while the claim might lead you to believe that corn oil is a "good" choice for health, you would actually have learned nothing about its properties relative to any other vegetable oil.

Similarly, there is sufficient latitude in the regulations for claims about ingredients, fat content, or calorie content, that many of these can be misleading. Rather than try to know every clever labeling strategy, you simply need to know which products are good choices. Once you have constructed a diet based mostly on healthful choices in every food category, you become more or less immune to misleading messages. (See Section IV, Food Label Guide)

Obstacle/Opportunity 8: Food Supply Globalization

The production and distribution of food has been transformed by technological advances. Food from anywhere in the world can be delivered to anywhere else in the world, any time. Affluent societies have more or less constant access to the food products of an entire planet.

There is obvious benefit in this, such as the availability of fresh produce in winter. But there is also disadvantage. Produce grown in another hemisphere is often harvested well before ripe, and may arrive less appetizing than local produce. And so much abundance, persistent throughout the year, may contribute to overeating.

The Then/Now Conflict

Agriculture was first developed some ten thousand years ago. Until then, during the preceding four million years of human and prehuman history, there was virtually no opportunity for humans to control the variety in their diets. Those foods available in a given place at a give time were what there was to eat. These foods varied with terrain, and climate, and season. Thus, there was variety over time, but the variety at any given time was subject to limits set by nature. Human ingenuity, applied to methods of food preservation and storage, allowed for some modest increase in dietary diversity, but the natural world set most of the limits. Until just the most recent decades, the food supply has been subject to natural limits. It no longer is.

Strategy

Access to a global food supply is a classic case of a potential obstacle to eating well that is clearly also an opportunity for eating well.

You, or your family, may like some, but not all, fruits or vegetables. In the past, your favorite produce would only be available seasonally. In most parts of the U.S., you can likely now find the produce you prefer any time of year. If so, you have a helpful means of maintaining a generous intake of the most health-promoting foods. Identify those varieties of vegetables and fruits you and your family will eat, then try to find an area market that makes them available all year long.

Bear in mind, however, that produce from halfway around the world may not have the vine-ripened flavor of local produce and you and your family may not realize how delicious some fruits and vegetables can be. Tomatoes, for example, taste completely different when ripened on the vine than when picked for shipping while still unripe. Even as you try to benefit from a year-round supply of produce, be sure to experience the best of local produce as a way of reminding yourself, and your family, that fruits and vegetables can truly be a delicious, as well as nutritious, component of the diet.

Finally, you will want to identify the nutritionally best products within each "category" of food, such as dressings, spreads, cereals, breads, soups, sauces, etc., and stick with them. Detailed guidance for finding preferred brands and products is provided in Section IV. Naturally, you have much more choice, and are much more likely to find products with both excellent nutrition and excellent taste, when you have access to products from around the globe. The modern food supply delivers this access to your supermarket

Obstacle/Opportunity 9: Inconvenience Involved in Finding, Ordering, or Preparing Nutritious Foods

There are two things that come very naturally when choosing foods. One is to eat what tastes good, and the other is to eat what's readily available. When those two characteristics come together, when tasty food is convenient food, it makes for considerable temptation. And if, as you try to improve your nutritional health, you not only have to limit your intake of some of your favorite foods, but also have to work twice as hard to find the new alternatives, you might very well get tired of the whole thing!

Today's nutritional environment, in which fatty, sugary, processed food abounds, represents a considerable obstacle to eating well. But this very same environment also abounds in opportunities to eat well; you simply need to know where, and how, to look.

Strategy

Combine your knowledge of a health-promoting dietary pattern with food label interpretation and good shopping skills, and you will start to find shopping for healthful foods far less challenging.

Once you get used to your new shopping pattern, all of the inconvenience goes away. You simply shop for the things you are used to, as you have always done. The difference is, now the things you are used to are promoting your health, controlling your weight, and lowering your cholesterol, blood sugar, or blood pressure, instead of doing just the opposite!

The same principles apply to cooking and eating out. Nutritious cooking is only inconvenient if you don't know how to do it! Once you learn what ingredients, techniques, and recipes to use, healthful food preparation is no longer inconvenient—it simply becomes the way you cook. Tips for stocking a health-promoting pantry are provided in Section IV, which also provides a meal planner, ingredient substitutions, and cooking methods.

The skills needed for choosing restaurants and eateries, and interpreting menus, are addressed in Step 6, and in Section IV. By using some simple strategies to find the right food choices, you can combine healthful eating at home, with comparably healthful eating out.

Fundamentally, the environment is neither convenient nor inconvenient when it comes to eating well. There are obstacles to eating well that will make doing so inconvenient if you run into them. There are opportunities for eating well that will make doing so very convenient, if you know where to find them.

Obstacle/Opportunity 10
Internet Use & Video Games

The less physical activity one does each day, the fewer calories required to maintain weight. For this reason, the combination of television viewing, Internet use, and computer games is thought to be a significant contributor to the modern obesity epidemic.

Strategy

The minimum level of moderate physical activity recommended for long-term health promotion is thirty minutes per day, most days of the week. Keeping this in mind is a useful way of gauging whether you, and/or your children, might be doing too little physically active recreation.

Set Limits on Physically Inactive Fun

No matter how much "fun" you or your kids have watching television, surfing the Net, or playing video games, limit these activities to certain days and/or hours. The strategy is quite similar to setting a limit on money you will spend in a casino, or at cards. These activities can be very costly if these limits are ignored, but are reasonable fun when the limits are respected. Sedentary recreations can also be fun, and harmless, if held at reasonable levels.

Look for all the opportunities in a typical week to replace inactive with active leisure time. If trying to increase the activity level of your children, one of the best approaches is to set an example they can follow. Choose from walking, biking, hiking, dancing, skiing, swimming, in-line skating, soccer, baseball, basketball, football, boating, landscaping, gardening, and countless other activities to find some ways in which you and your family can enjoy sharing in some physical exertion.

Exercising Love & Discipline

To the extent that peer influences are encouraging your children to spend more and more time online or playing video games, address these directly. Young people in the U.S. and other industrialized countries are increasingly overweight and out of shape. Without being critical, you can help your kids understand that this particular peer influence places them at risk of these conditions. Let them partake, but set reasonable limits. As you do in so many ways being a parent, combine love, support, and understanding with setting limits and discipline so you can protect your child's fun, as well as their health.

Obstacle/Opportunity 11: Misleading Menus

When you eat outside of the home, you are dependent on information provided by others to know anything about the nutritional properties of the food. If, for example, you are at a restaurant or diner, you may try to choose among the more healthful items based on the information available on the menu.

Unfortunately, you really can't make assumptions about nutrition based on the name of a dish. A vegetarian dish, for example, may not be lower in fat than a meat dish. A meal based on pasta, or chicken, or fish, may or may not offer better nutrition than alternatives. It all depends on the combination of ingredients the dish contains.

And many of these ingredients tend to go unmentioned. A sauce based on cream may not be listed. Cheese, or croutons, in a salad may not be mentioned. The ingredients, sauces, spreads, and dressings that add the most in terms of calories, or fat, may come as a surprise when the dish arrives. If you eat out a lot, being alert to the deficiencies in most menus is an important challenge to address.

Strategy

Recall that it is the overall pattern of the diet that matters, not a particular food, or meal, or even day. If you usually eat at home, and if your nutrition is generally good, you may choose to eat out occasionally just for the pleasure of it, and not to worry about nutrition. This is reasonable.

If, however, you eat out a lot, you will need to admit that what you eat when you eat out has a significant impact on the overall quality of your diet. To eat well under these circumstances requires that you be adequately informed. Start by identifying eating places convenient to you that offer nutritious options. If a particular restaurant or fast-food outlet specializes in high-fat, high-calorie foods, it is best to find alternative eating places.

Find the Best, Then Choose the Best

Once you identify the best places, try to identify the best menu choices. In this context, "best" means those dishes most compatible with the recommended dietary pattern. Dishes based on grains and vegetables are generally good choices. Poultry and fish are generally preferable to red meat. Grilling, baking, and broiling are generally preferable to frying.

But often, you need to go further. And here is where you need to establish an arrangement that works for you. It's no fun to interrogate your waiter or waitress when you are eating out! On the other hand, if you don't ask some questions, you may be very misled by the menu.

The Regular Customer

If you are eating in a restaurant you do, or will, eat in often, you should probably make a pretty thorough inquiry about the menu. Ask, in particular, about whether a dish is high in fat, and about cream, butter, and/or cheese in sauces, spreads, and dressings. In addition to learning about what is usually in the menu items, ask if it's possible to get items that are low in fat. A restaurant unwilling to accommodate your nutrition preferences may be a place you do not want to visit often. Once you identify the "preferred" menu items, and get to know the ways in which the chef or cook can modify dishes to suit your tastes, you have a good basis to make informed decisions. Use these insights to eat well while eating out.

If you are at a restaurant that you will not be visiting often, a less labor-intensive approach will likely make sense. You can simply indicate that you prefer to avoid, for example, food that is rich, and would like some advice about menu items relatively low in fat. You can identify specific items you would like to avoid—such as butter or cream—and again, ask for guidance. Just a few questions can help you know enough to make good choices.

Unless you have a particular health reason to emphasize the salt or sugar content of your food, focus on the fat content when you review a menu, or discuss dishes with a waiter or waitress. For the most part, relatively low-fat dishes will be the ones best suited to a healthy way of eating.

There is no reason why eating out should not offer the combination of convenience, fun, and good nutrition. But for that to happen, you need to take control. Avoid assumptions, and remember that the nutritional environment will not take care of you—you need to take care of yourself!

Obstacle/Opportunity 12: School Policies

In an ideal world, the places we congregate would all reinforce health-promoting behaviors. This should be especially true of places children congregate, schools being the best example. But even school lunch pro-grams meeting federal guidelines provide children access to a wide array of highly processed, high-fat, high-sugar, high-salt foods. And, because children receiving a nutritionally balanced meal are not necessarily chil-dren eating a nutritionally balanced meal, the availability of these less-than-ideal choices often contributes to less than ideal dietary patterns. Additionally, many schools house vending machines, or even fast-food restaurants, giving children and adolescents convenient access to tempt-ing, but nutritionally poor, choices. And finally, pressures on schools to conform to state or federal curricular guidelines are increasingly squeez-ing physical education, and even recess, out of the typical day.

Strategy

There is increasing interest in, and attention to, school policies among public health personnel devoted to nutrition and physical activity. This attention is particularly intense because of the clearly worsening epi-demic of childhood obesity and diabetes in the United States. As a result, policy changes with the potential to improve the influence of schools on dietary and activity patterns may be coming to a neighbor-hood near you soon. We hope so! But, if your children are subject to adverse health exposures now, it's best not to hope for, and wait for, policy changes. You can take action now.

Family Matters

First, make nutrition, physical activity, and health family matters, not just a personal matter for you. Your own efforts to achieve weight con-trol and nutritional health will be much easier if you are supported by the members of your household. And by getting involved in your efforts, your family members will get similar benefits for themselves. Everyone wins.

Let your children know that you care about their health, and that you therefore care about their diet and activity. What you say will of course be most impactful if you are setting, or working to set, a good example.

If your children are old enough, talk to them about the school day and the school food. Inquire about the choices they make, and discuss

---

Katz' Tales...

Valerie, age seven, is in first grade. Like the rest of us Katzes, she eats well. And because that's the *way* it is in our home, she thinks that it's simply the way things should be—with that single-mindedness only kids have.

So is she tempted by the foods she encounters in school? Apparently not—in fact, if anything, she's a little too self-righteous (we're working on that!).

Mom—you know what? My teacher, Mrs. Connor, sometimes eats doughnuts! Can you believe it? But she's a very good teacher...

---

alternatives. They may benefit, as you do, from taking food with them each day. Alternatively, they may be able, with guidance, to make better choices from among the selection available at school. Help your children find ways, and times, to be physically active. And whenever possible, join in, for their benefit, as well as your own.

Take Nutrition Concerns to the Big Cheeses
Young children will of course be less capable of assessing their school exposures, or of compensating for them if they are not ideal. So, you need to go over their heads! Ask about nutrition and physical activity in school at open houses, and parent-teacher conferences. Let the school administration know that these are things you care about, and what your wishes are. These issues should be priorities for all parents and all schools in the U.S. because obesity and diabetes are a very serious threat to our kids.

There's No Place Like Home
Finally, remember that the greatest influence on your children is you. If you establish healthful eating and activity patterns at home, your children will carry these influences and examples with them out into the world. Even if exposures outside of home introduce some "junk" food into the diets of your children, they will tolerate this far better if their

home nutritional environment is a safe one. In the long run, the foods of home leave a strong and influential impression on most of us.

Obstacle/Opportunity 13: Sedentary Pastimes

Singer Paul Simon says this is the age of "miracle and wonder." Many of the wonders of modern society take the form of technology that reduces the need for physical work, and creates opportunity for sedentary leisure pursuits.

Probably the single most important product of technology to reduce leisure-time activity is the television. Television viewing is considered by the Centers for Disease Control and Prevention (CDC) to be one of the leading risk factors for obesity in childhood. Internet use and video games further increase the hours per week spent being inactive. Snowmobiles often replace snowshoes and cross-country skis. All-terrain vehicles replace walking shoes. Jet skis may replace water skis. Increasingly, even fairly active leisure pursuits are being made less vigorous by technology; you can be a real outdoorsman, and never break a sweat!

The math here is very simple. If physical activity on the job, at home, and in the yard is reduced or eliminated by technology; if hours formerly spent in active leisure pursuits are now spent watching television or on the Internet; and if even fairly active hobbies are less vigorous than they once were, the total reduction in average energy expenditure (physical activity) is tremendous. The end result? The couch potato!

Strategy

The role of nutrition in health cannot really be separated from the role of physical activity. How many calories are "too many" depends in part on physical activity level, and muscle mass. Basal metabolic rate, the primary determinant of calories needed to maintain weight, is itself influenced by activity, muscle mass, and conditioning. To achieve lasting nutritional health and weight control simply requires routine physical activity.

Learning to Want What You Need

If you are tempted to spend many hours each week watching television, using the Internet, or engaging in some other sedentary pastime, consider setting a limit to these activities, and protecting time for more

---

Hills: Pain, or Gain?

Ellen, forty-two, has the good fortune of living in a beautiful neighborhood. There is a wonderful, quiet loop, several miles long, on country roads that makes for an ideal walk. The problem? Ellen hates hills, and there are two. Neither is a mountain, but it's only fair to admit they aren't exactly mole hills, either!

We talked about why she hates these hills—and it's mostly because they make her breathless. They also cause a burning in her legs. On the other hand, she is especially interested in toning her legs. So we talked about the message in that burning. It's a sign that she's conditioning the very muscles she wants to condition. And the breathlessness? Perhaps a sign she's going too fast, but also clear evidence she's conditioning her heart.

I can't say Ellen has learned to love those hills…but they have come to an understanding. She's slowed down a bit, for less pain. But she also focuses on the benefits so that the "gain" keeps her going! And with her improving fitness, those hills keep getting smaller all the time.

---

active pursuits. Use the goal of thirty minutes or more of moderate activity on most days as a way of gauging your balance between physically active, and inactive, hobbies. If you are very committed to sedentary pastimes, look for ways to build physical activity into your work day, or compensate by exercising at a fixed time each day.

Be sure to recognize the value in physical activity as a way of reinforcing it. Whenever you walk, push, or carry instead of sit, or ride, feel the muscles you are using and consider the wide array of health benefits. Calories burned. Muscles conditioned. Metabolic rate increased.

Technological advances are dangerously seductive because we wind up feeling as if we should, or must, make use of them to keep up with the times. Be forewarned, and thus forearmed, against the dangers of too much reliance on technology for play, as well as for work. Rely on your own muscles instead, at least some of the time, and they will pay you back with abundant health benefits.

Obstacle/Opportunity 14: Suburban Design Issues

Perhaps nothing represents the hazards of the modern environment quite so well as suburbia. Cities are so densely clustered, with residential and commercial areas intermingled, that they allow for many routine chores to be completed on foot. Rural areas often are associated with outdoor activities that increase physical exertion. Suburbs combine the amenities and conveniences of cities, with distances that often prevent reaching destinations on foot.

Thus, the design of suburbs in the U.S. makes those of us who live in them extremely dependent on our cars. With busy lives, if we do not find time to be active during the routine part of the day, many of us have difficulty finding the time, energy, or inclination to exercise at the end of the day, or first thing in the morning. So the car dependence associated with suburban design is directly associated with low levels of physical activity.

But the hazards of suburbia don't stop there. Fast-food restaurants abound. And because everyone spends so much time in cars, the environment has been redesigned to accommodate the needs of cars (not necessarily the same needs as the people driving them!). Drive-through restaurants, banks, and businesses lead to reduced physical activity. The types of restaurants that have drive-throughs are generally serving the types of food a health-promoting diet should minimize. Achieving health and weight control in this setting is a challenge, to be sure! But like most challenges, it is one that you can meet if appropriately prepared.

Strategy

Strategies for meeting the challenges of suburban living, and for turning obstacles into opportunities, vary in intensity. Let's start with some modest approaches. If you have a choice between shopping at multiple sites and driving to each, or shopping in a mall that allows access to all of the stores you need, choose the mall. Walking is beneficial whether indoors or out, and while they may not be so great for your wallet or pocketbook, malls do make good indoor walking sites. Take advantage of a trip to a big mall to walk all around, rather than directly to the stores you need, whenever your schedule permits.

Small Steps That Add Up

Look for the parking space farthest from, rather than closest to, the store or building you are about to enter; if you get the space farthest away, you win! What you win is the benefit of some additional walking time. Be practical about this, of course. If the weather is terrible, or you have small children, or too much to carry, that parking space right next to the entrance starts looking pretty irresistible! As with all of your efforts to achieve health and weight control, decide where to set limits you consider reasonable. There is no benefit in pushing beyond that point, because you will likely get aggravated and give up! Instead, make changes you can live with, and add to them gradually.

Whenever possible, avoid the use of your car. For some chores, you may have a choice between use of your car and walking, or use of your car and biking. Try to allocate time to use your feet or bike. Even if you do this only periodically, it can contribute to your well-being.

Be creative in finding opportunities for physical activity in the suburban environment. Try to make good use of parks, greenways, bike paths, ball fields, and backyards. If your health permits, turn the very features of suburbia into opportunities to be active. Use a push-mower rather than a ride-on lawn mower. Use a rake rather than a leaf-blower. Shovel your driveway, rather than having it plowed. Gather firewood in your backyard, rather than buying it. In these and other ways, you can turn tending to your suburban home into varied opportunities for physical activity.

Drive by Instead of Through

Resist drive-throughs whenever possible. In particular, try to avoid drive-through, fast-food restaurants that combine inactivity with poor nutrition. If you'll be in your car for a while, pack up healthful snacks for yourself, and if they're with you, for your kids. Try, when the weather is good and your busy schedule permits, to view parking and getting out of the car as an opportunity to stretch and exercise your legs a bit, rather than an inconvenience.

Your Neighborhood, Your Batch of Strategies

Once you have started to size up your personal environment, pull from among the many strategies in this book, or others you devise yourself, those that are most relevant and helpful. Design a personalized batch of strategies that matches your environment. As you do, remain alert to those barriers that continue to get in your way, or new ones that come along. Build on your successes, and view unresolved challenges as opportunities.

Obstacle/Opportunity 15
Weight-Loss Industry Claims/Unregulated Products

In response to the ever-worsening epidemic of obesity in the United States and other industrialized countries, an industry valued in the billions of dollars has developed to generate weight-loss products and services. This industry is responsible for adding many new supplements to the market each year, and for millions and millions of dollars in advertising on radio, television, the Internet, and in print. For most of us, this results in a nearly continuous barrage of weight-loss industry messages, many if not most of which are unsubstantiated, inaccurate, misleading, or in the extreme, deceitful.

Strategy

There are two simple elements to the strategy required for dealing effectively and successfully with the barrage of weight-loss propaganda. The first is to invoke the business adage *caveat emptor*, or "buyer beware" as discussed earlier. Recall that anyone selling something is, well, selling something! That in and of itself does not discredit the product, but it does offer a reason other than your well-being why the product might be promoted!

Second, be honest with yourself about your state of both need and naïveté. If you are trying to control your weight, and have years of frustration and limited if any success to show for it, you have certainly created a sellers' market! You are in no position to drive a hard bargain, demand evidence, or resist a well-spun tale. You are, in a word, desperate for something that will, or even could, work. Recognize that as long as this state persists, you are every salesman's dream come true!

The Weight of Evidence

The steps beyond this are more involved, but also, ultimately more rewarding. One is to become knowledgeable about the causes of weight gain, and responsible means of weight loss. By doing so, you acquire a certain savvy about weight loss that allows you either to avoid commercial products altogether, or choose them carefully. You may not, in other words, find your way to thinness right away, but you will have some sense of both where you are, and where you want to go, allowing you to tell good directions from bad.

The most definitive defense against discreditable weight-loss products or advice is, of course, weight loss! Once you are securely on the way to a healthful relationship with your diet, one that leads to better weight control and improved health, you will not be easily tempted to follow misleading advice toward undesired destinations.

There Are No Secrets

Several other issues are important to consider. If a weight-loss product were truly effective, the medical and nutrition communities would know about it. Naturally, clinicians and dietitians are eager for safe and effective products that can aid weight-control efforts by patients and clients, and have no reason to dispute legitimate claims. Those suppliers claiming to have uncovered some truth only they know are much more likely to be harboring a false claim only they are interested in making. Truths stand up quite well to the light of public exposure and professional inquiry. When it is "privileged" information that sounds too good to be true, it almost certainly is.

Also worth considering is that there are some products and services of true potential value. As you learn to be a knowledgeable consumer, you want to be skeptical, but not cynical.

The evidence of effectiveness, in terms of sustainable weight loss, is limited for even the most legitimate of interventions. To some extent, choosing a program or service that's both reasonable, and tailored to your needs, may be a useful adjunct to your weight-control efforts. A consideration of reasonable products and programs is provided in Section IV.

If It's the Environment...

...THAT MAKES WEIGHT control and eating well difficult, then it really is the environment that should be changed, not you! The skills and strategies of the *way to eat* allow you to navigate around the many obstacles the modern environment places between you and health, weight control, and happiness with food.

But the *way* would be easier and more direct if the environment were changed into one that made eating well and being physically active easy, commonplace, and always accessible.

There are ways you can help change the world. When the going gets tough, the tough may get going, but the smart also look for ways to make the going less tough! Our suggestion is that you be both tough, and smart. Even as you gain the knowledge, power, skills, and strategies to work your way successfully through the modern nutritional environment, you should be aware, and take advantage, of the many opportunities you have to influence the conditions of that world.

Does your town or neighborhood provide you with safe, well-lit places to walk or exercise? Is there a park? Do your schools have vending machines filled with "junk" food to entice your children? Does the area supermarket offer the products and brands you want? Does your workplace provide access to healthful foods? Is there time during the work day for a walk? When you go to a fast-food restaurant or cafeteria, do you know the nutritional content of the foods you are ordering?

The answers to these questions suggest actions you can take—as a citizen, a taxpayer, a parent, or a constituent—to help change the world. Let your local politicians, and those running for office in your town, know that opportunities to eat well and be physically active matter to you. Use parent-teacher conferences, school assemblies, meetings of the local school board, or meetings of parent-teacher organizations (PTA and PTO) to ask about school nutrition policies, and let your views be known. Find others who share your views—in clubs or congregations, classes or the workplace—and express your opinions in a common voice. Remember our good fortune in living in a democracy; when enough of us care about an issue, we really can change the world! Below is a list of some of the changes in policies, programs, and the environment we recommend you support.

Recommended Changes in Policies, Programs, and Practices that Shape the Nutritional Environment

Neighborhoods
Sidewalks should be available.

Safe bicycle paths should be available.

Parks and recreational facilities should be available, accessible, and safe.

Urban development plans should include creating opportunities for walking and biking.

Schools
Vending machines should be banned, or should provide healthful choices.

Sodas in schools should be replaced with bottled waters or natural juices.

Cafeterias should provide healthful and appealing foods.

All children should receive skilled instruction in healthful eating, and its importance.

Physical education should be mandatory, and should contribute to fitness.

Schools should provide opportunities for physically active recreation after-hours.

Work places Stairs should be accessible, well-lit, and inviting.

Breaks for walking or other physical activity should be routine.

Healthful eating should be encouraged; as appropriate, healthful food choices should be made available on-site.

Supermarkets Information should be available on-site to guide healthful shopping.

Dietitians should be on-site at certain times to answer questions, indicate preferred products, and help improve overall nutrition.

Distances walked through the store should be posted to help point out the benefits of physical activity in routine chores.

Hospitals & other institutions Healthful food should be provided; what is "preached" should be practiced.

The nutritional composition of meals should be provided.

Restaurants All fast-food restaurants should post calorie and nutrient content of meals along with prices.

All restaurants should have nutrient composition of dishes available on request.

All restaurants should provide nutritious options.

Incentives for the creation of "healthy" fast-food restaurants and eateries should be provided by communities.

Other

All health insurers should reimburse for professional nutrition and physical activity counseling by dietitians and health-care professionals.

Health insurers and/or employers should contribute toward the cost of home exercise equipment or gym membership.

Modest taxes on soda or "junk" foods (e.g., one cent per can of soda) should be used to raise funds for nutrition education, build physical activity facilities, conduct social marketing campaigns for nutritious eating, and other related purposes.

Skilled daycare should be available at gyms, aerobics classes, etc., so that parents with young children can partake.

Food advertising should be regulated so that the nutritional content is described accurately.

Many of these suggestions are courtesy of: Nestle, Marion, and Jacobson, Michael F., "Halting the Obesity Epidemic: A Public Health Policy Approach." *Public Health Reports.* 2000; 115:12–24.

Section Four:

Paving the Way...
to Eat

In Sections I–III, our focus has been on you—your ability to find and follow the *way*. Now, we turn to the *way* itself. In its twelve parts, Section IV gives you the detailed, practical information and resources you need to apply every strategy offered in the prior Steps to the places you shop and eat out; the foods you buy; the recipes and ingredients you use; the meals you prepare; the pantry you stock; the menus and labels you encounter; the places you work, study, and live. Ultimately, it is not ideas about eating, but the actual foods, and meals, and snacks we do eat that determine our nutritional health. Think of these resources as the very paving stones of the *way*, as important as your knowledge of the route and your commitment to following it.

Use these resource materials to translate advice and strategies into behaviors that are a part of your everyday life. As you do, please remember that every new skill you acquire and every step you take that brings you closer to your nutrition and health goals is a success. We wish you the very best of eating, and of health: *bon appetit* and *bon voyage!*

Section Four
Table of Contents

Resource 1: *The Way to Eat Well: Basic Principles & General Guidelines*

This entry provides the recommended *way to eat* dietary pattern, both in terms of nutritional composition, and food choices, along with the basic philosophy about diet and health on which these recommendations are based.

The Way to Eat Philosophy

In the modern nutritional environment, so at odds with our ancient metabolic drives and adaptations, eating a healthful diet and controlling your weight are challenging. The adoption of any new behavior, or the application of any new skill or strategy that improves your diet, should be considered a success. A healthful diet and its benefits will likely be achieved in steps. Each step along the way is commendable. Make sure you give yourself appropriate credit; we do!

You do not directly control your weight, your cholesterol, or your blood pressure. You do, ultimately, have control over the way you choose to eat, and your physical activity pattern. These, in turn, influence your health, and your weight. Whatever your health and weight goals, we encourage you to focus on the behaviors you control, and measure your success based on them. Health improvement and weight control will follow the adoption of health-promoting behaviors. But even if you eat very well, and are physically active, you may not reach your "fantasy" weight, or avoid a need for medication to lower your cholesterol. You might...but you might not. If you don't, we support the adage that you should strive for the strength to change the things you can, the patience to accept the things you cannot, and the wisdom to tell the two apart.

Another important consideration is all the ways learning to eat well is like learning a new language. When you don't speak a language, everything about even a simple sentence is confusing. Once you are fluent in a language, everything about it is suddenly easy—it becomes second nature. In learning to eat well, too, even simple recommendations depend on not one, but many skills. To shop well, you need to be able to interpret food labels. To cook well, you need to shop well. And so on. Our approach to this issue is on the one hand to focus on each individual skill, strategy, or fact you need, and on the other hand to acknowledge the interdependence of many skills, strategies, and facts. Keep in mind that even babies learn new languages just by hearing them, and that once you speak a language, everything about it is suddenly easy. You don't need to think about the rules of grammar to speak English; you just know how to speak it. Traveling along the *way to eat* will make you just as fluent in good eating. Just don't expect to find everything you need to know in any one step along the way—it is spread out all along the journey.

Finally, we reiterate the fundamental premise on which all of our guidance is based: there is a *way to eat* that is consistent with health and longevity and weight control. Alternatives to a prudent dietary pattern offer a choice between weight control and health, and ultimately deliver neither! You probably know this already, because you've likely been there, done that! We reject this choice altogether; the same way of eating offers both benefits. Eating well is a lifelong activity; it is not six weeks of "dieting" intended to reduce your belt or dress size. The challenge of eating well is about *how*; we truly do already know *what*. To achieve this diet, the "obstacles" of the modern nutritional environment can and should be seen as opportunities to develop and apply the skills and strategies needed to keep moving steadily along your *way*.

Recommended Nutritional Composition
of the Way to Eat

Nutrient Class/Nutrient	Recommended Intake
Carbohydrate, predominately complex	Approximately 55–60% of total calories
Fiber, both soluble and insoluble	At least 25 grams per day, with additional potential benefit from up to 50 grams per day
Protein, predominantly plant-based sources	Up to 20% of total calories
Total Fat	
Types of Fat	Not more than 30%, and preferably 20–25% of total calories
Monounsaturated Fat	10% of total calories
Polyunsaturated Fat	10% of total calories
Omega-3 and Omega-6 Fat	1:1 to 1:4 ratio
Saturated Fat & Trans Fat (partially hydrogenated fat)	Ideally, less than 5% of total calories
Sugar	Less than 10% of total calories
Sodium	Up to 2,400 mg per day
Cholesterol	Less than 300 mg a day
Water	8 glasses a day/64 oz/2 liters
Alcohol, moderate intake if desired	Up to one drink a day for women Up to two drinks a day for men
Calorie Level	Adequate to achieve & maintain a healthy weight
Physical Activity / Exercise	Daily moderate activity for 30 minutes/Strength training twice weekly

Recommended Foods & Overall Dietary Pattern

Food Group	Foods to Choose[†]
Whole Grains	Choose at least 7 to 8 servings a day of whole-grain breads, cereals, and grains with 2 or more grams of fiber per serving. Include oatmeal, oat bran, brown and wild rice varieties, semolina and whole-wheat pasta, couscous, barley, and bulgur wheat.
Fruits	Choose 4 to 5 servings a day from a rainbow of colors, especially deep yellow, orange, and red: berries, apples, oranges, apricots, melons, mangos, etc. Select from fresh, frozen, canned packed in juice, and dried varieties. Buy locally grown in season whenever possible.
Vegetables	Choose 4 to 5 servings a day from a rainbow of colors, especially deep yellow, orange, red, and leafy green: yellow, red, and green bell peppers; squash, carrots, tomatoes, spinach, sweet potatoes, broccoli, kale, Swiss chard, Brussels sprouts, eggplant, etc. Select from fresh, frozen, and canned varieties but be mindful of the higher sodium content of canned. Buy locally grown in season whenever possible.
Beans & Legumes	Include 3 to 4 times a week. Beans and legumes make a good alternative to meat. Include a variety of beans and legumes in your diet: black, red, kidney, white, cannellini, garbanzo (chick pea), navy, pinto, lentils, split peas, black-eyed peas, soy.

Food Group	Foods to Choose[†]	(continued)
Fish*(& Seafood)	Include as often as 3 to 4 times a week if desired. Fish is generally an excellent, lean source of high-quality protein, and several varieties (e.g., tuna, salmon, mackerel, halibut, and cod) are excellent sources of Omega-3 fatty acids. Seafood, such as shrimp and scallops, tends to be relatively high in cholesterol but is low in fat, and also a good source of omega-3 fatty acids.	
Chicken & Turkey*	Include up to 1 to 2 times a week. Skinless breast meat is preferred.	
Lean Beef, Pork, Lamb*	Moderate your intake of meat, working toward a goal of roughly 1 to 2 meat-based meals per week, or 4 to 8 per month, if desired. Select lean meats preferentially; the loin and round cuts are the leanest.	
Milk & Cheese*	Choose at least 2 servings a day from fat-free, skim, or low-fat versions.	
Vegetable Oils & Other Added Fats	Choose monounsaturated and polyunsaturated sources daily, but use in very small amounts: olive oil, canola oil, olives, avocados, almond butter, and peanut butter.	
Nuts & Seeds	Include 4 to 5 times a week in small amounts of unsalted raw or dry roasted types: almonds, walnuts, pistachios, peanuts, pecans, cashews, soy nuts, sunflower seeds, pumpkin seeds, sesame seeds. Mix 1 tablespoon of ground flaxseed daily into other cooked foods.	

Food Group	Foods to Choose†	(continued)
Eggs*	Up to 2 egg yolks per week on average. Preferably, choose an omega-3 fatty acid enriched brand.	
Sweets	Use in moderation. Choose low or nonfat varieties whenever reasonable.	

*Optional items. Well-balanced vegetarian and vegan diets are wholly compatible with the *way to eat*. See Resource 2 for meat alternatives. Note that fish is recommended for particular health benefits; flaxseeds, and/or an omega-3 fatty acid supplement are especially recommended to those who don't eat fish.

† See Resource 9 for serving size guidelines.

Resource 2: *The Way to Navigate the Nutritional Environment*

These entries address important "exposures" in the modern nutritional environment, and provide guidance in interpreting and/or dealing successfully with them.

Alternatives to Meat

Foods are good alternatives to meat if they substitute well for the valuable protein in meat, and if they replace the role of meat in recipes in terms of taste, texture, and heartiness, or both. Reducing meat in the diet generally helps to reduce total fat and cholesterol intake. There are potential environmental benefits of less meat consumption by our society as well, discussed in such books as: John Robbin's *The Food Revolution: How Your Diet Can Help Save Your Life and the World*; and Frances Moore Lappe's *Diet for a Small Planet*.

- **Beans:** excellent source of high quality protein with added benefit of fiber and many nutrients; provide complete protein when combined with vegetables or grains
- **Eggplant:** versatile vegetable for cooking with a hearty texture and "meaty" taste
- **Egg White:** versatile in cooking, adds complete protein
- **Falafel:** made from chick peas, a kind of legume; excellent source of protein, nutrients, and fiber; hearty and satisfying
- **Lentils:** available in several varieties, add a nutty and/or meaty taste and texture; excellent source of protein, nutrients, and soluble fiber
- **Nuts & Seeds:** can be added to many recipes, or eaten in snacks, to replace protein from meat; also rich in many nutrients, fiber, and often essential fatty acids
- **Portobello Mushrooms:** taste and texture is meaty; when cooked and seasoned, good substitute for beef in sandwiches
- **Tofu:** made from soybeans; versatile in cooking and baking; provides high-quality protein, essential fatty acids, and many other nutrients; comes in marinated,

ready-to-eat varieties that make an excellent substitute for sandwich meats

- **Veggie Burgers:** available in many varieties (see Resource 4), some more nutritious than others; generally made from combinations of vegetables and grains that offer considerable nutritional advantages over ground beef

Energy Density of Macronutrient Classes

Nutrient Class	Calorie Content	Comments
Carbohydrate	4kcal/gram	Although all carbohydrate provides 4kcal/gram, not all carbohydrate is created equal! Complex carbohydrate sources are high in fiber, which is indigestible, and free of calories. If fiber is high in a product, it will lower the calorie content for any given portion size. Additionally, high-fiber foods tend to be more filling (i.e., they have a higher satiety index).
Protein	4kcal/gram	Protein sources are more valuable if they provide the amino acids and protein building blocks our bodies need most. The best sources of protein include egg white, fish, poultry, soybeans, meat, and beans and lentils. Protein has a higher satiety index than fat, and a slightly higher satiety index than high-fiber carbohydrate.
Fat	9kcal/gram	Fat is the most energy dense, and least satiating, of the macronutrients. It therefore tends to contribute the most to "excess" calories.
Alcohol	7kcal/gram	Alcohol is a frequently overlooked source of calories.

Fat Substitutes

- The principal reason for fat substitution is to reduce total fat and calorie intake.
- The available evidence suggests that fat substitutes are generally effective at reducing fat intake, but not necessarily at reducing calorie intake, because people often make up for the removed fat calories by eating more calories from other sources.
- There are three basic categories of fat replacers: fat mimetics, fat substitutes, and low-calorie fats. Fat mimetics are nonfat food items that replace fats; mimic the properties fats confer including effects on flavor and palatability, creaminess, and mouth feel; and add fewer calories than the fats they replace. Examples include starches, cellulose, pectin, proteins, dextrins, polydextrose, and other products.
- Fat mimetics are often useful in desserts and spreads, and are generally of less use in foods that require frying or other high-temperature preparation. Fat mimetics range from 0 to 4 kcal per gram.
- Low-calorie fats are fat molecules (triglycerides) modified to deliver less than the 9 kcal per gram of most naturally occurring fats. Commercially produced low-calorie fats are poorly absorbed due to the attachment of fatty acids of varying chain lengths to glycerol; the calorie content of such products as Caprenin (Proctor & Gamble) and Salatrim (Nabisco) is approximately 5 kcal per gram.
- Soluble fibers used as fat substitutes confer health benefits independent of fat replacement, such as cholesterol reduction and reduced insulin release. For some individuals, processed, fat-reduced foods could become a significant source of soluble fiber.
- The most studied fat substitute to date is a sucrose polyester, Olestra, developed by Proctor & Gamble and marketed as Olean. Because it is essentially indigestible, Olestra passes through the gastrointestinal tract carrying fat-soluble micronutrients with it. Approved by the FDA

for use in snack foods, Olestra is controversial because of the potential for both gastrointestinal upset and the leaching of these fat-soluble nutrients.

Olestra decreases absorption of vitamins A, D, E, and K, but this effect is at least partially compensated by the fortification of Olestra-containing foods with fat-soluble vitamins. Most evidence suggests that Olestra-containing snack foods, consumed under ordinary circumstances, do not produce any more gastrointestinal symptoms than standard products.

- A variety of products derived from alterations of fat molecules are under development.
- For now, limited use of products that use fat substitutes seems quite reasonable, but reliance on fat substitutes as a primary strategy to reduce fat or calorie intake cannot be recommended.

Fatty Acid Facts

Category of Fatty Acid	Food Sources	Comments
Monounsaturated	Olives, nuts, avocados, olive oil, canola oil	Monounsaturated fatty acids are a mainstay in the "Mediterranean" diet and are associated with health benefits. Shifting fat calories from saturated and trans fat to monounsaturated fat is recommended.
Polyunsaturated	**Omega-6** Nuts, seeds, grains, leafy vegetables soybeans, dairy products, corn oil, safflower oil, soybean oil	Omega-6 fatty acids are essential to good health. However, the modern diet tends to provide much more access to omega-6 than to omega-3 fatty acids, and an imbalance is bad for health.

Category of Fatty Acid	Food Sources	Comments
		(continued)
		Prioritize sources of omega- 3 fatty acids to approximate a 1:1 ratio for these two important types of fat.
Omega-3	Cold-water fish (mackerel, salmon, cod, halibut)	Omega-3 fatty acids are essential to health, and tend to be deficient in most modern diets. Eating fish regularly, adding flaxseeds or flaxseed oil to the diet, and/or using a fish-oil supplement are recommended to create a balance between omega-3 and omega-6 fatty acids.
Saturated	Meat, poultry, whole-fat dairy, coconut oil, palm oil, palm kernel oil	Saturated fat raises cholesterol and heart disease risk, and tends to be excessive in the modern diet. An effort should be made to reduce or avoid the sources of saturated fat.
Trans	Processed foods containing partially hydrogenated oils	Trans fat, produced when naturally unsaturated fats are "saturated" with hydrogen, has the same adverse health effects as saturated fat; sources of trans fat in the diet should be reduced or avoided.

Fiber Facts

A high intake of dietary fiber offers a range of health benefits, and can help control weight. We recommend an intake level of at least 25 to 30 grams, and preferably as much as 50 grams per day for every 2,000 kcal. You will naturally tend to have a high intake of fiber if your overall pattern of eating is, as recommended, based mostly on whole grains, fruits, and vegetables, all of which are high in fiber.

- Fiber is by definition indigestible plant material, generally considered in the carbohydrate category because fiber comes from foods that are made up mostly of carbohydrate.
- There are two principal classes of fiber: soluble and insoluble.
- Soluble, or viscous, fiber dissolves in water; insoluble fiber does not.
- When soluble fiber dissolves, it forms a slurry in the gastrointestinal tract. This delays the absorption of glucose and fatty acids into the blood stream, lowering post-eating (postprandial) levels of glucose, triglycerides, other lipids, and insulin in the blood. This is thought to be the primary mechanism for the health benefits of soluble fiber.
- Soluble fiber eaten regularly can lower cholesterol and other lipids in the blood stream.
- Soluble fibers of relative importance include guar gum, psyllium, pectin, and ß-glucan.
- Insoluble fiber, or roughage, stimulates the gastrointestinal system, and speeds transit through the intestines. This is thought to be beneficial to intestinal health, possibly lowering the risk of colon cancer and other diseases of the bowel.
- Important insoluble fibers include lignins, celluloses, and hemicelluloses.
- Both categories of fiber may increase the satiety index of foods, leading to a sense of fullness that can help control appetite and reduce calorie intake.
- Because fiber is by definition "indigestible," it provides no calories.
- Dietary guidelines call for an intake of approximately 30 grams/day of total fiber, divided more or less evenly between soluble and insoluble fiber. We recommend at least 25 grams per 2,000 kcal, preferably closer to 50 grams.
- The average fiber intake of adults in the U.S. is about 12 grams per day, or less than half the recommended level.

- Fiber is especially beneficial if you have insulin resistance, high cholesterol, diabetes, constipation, or are trying to lose weight.
- The health benefits of fiber are generally unaffected by food preparation, cooking, and storage under normal conditions.

Foods That Are Rich in Fiber

Food	Amount	Energy (kcal)	Fiber (g)
Wheat bran (raw)	1 cup (58 g)	125	25
Oat bran (raw)	1 cup (94 g)	231	14.5
Bulgur wheat	1 cup (182 g), cooked	151	8.2
Raspberries	1 cup (123 g)	60	8.4
Barley, pearled	1 cup (157 g), cooked	193	6
Lentils	1 cup (198 g), cooked	230	15.6
Bread, whole wheat	1 slice (28 g)	69	2
Chick peas	1 cup (164 g)	269	12.5
Brown rice	1 cup (195 g), cooked	218	3.5
Apples	1 medium (138 g)	81	3.7
Pasta	1 cup (140 g), cooked	197	2.4
Carrots	1 medium (61 g)	26	1.8

* Insoluble fiber is abundant in whole grains, especially wheat; soluble fiber is abundant in fruits, oats, lentils, and beans.

* Values for all grains are reported for cooked portions unless otherwise stated.

* The nutrient composition of foods is obtained from the U.S.DA Nutrient database at: www.nal.usda.gov/fnic/foodcomp/Data/SR 14. Table adapted from: Katz, D.L., *Nutrition in Clinical Practice*. Philadelphia, PA: Lippincott Williams & Wilkins, 2000. Reprinted with permission of the publisher.

Foods to Limit

While the quality of your overall dietary pattern has a tremendous influence on your health, a single food, eaten from time to time, for the most part does not. So no food needs to be entirely excluded from your diet for you to eat well.

However, there are foods that tend to contribute a lot of saturated or trans fat, cholesterol, sugar, or salt to the average diet. The health threat of these foods is associated with the way they add up. For example:

Mr. M (a patient): "Doc, you said it's OK if I sometimes eat steak, right? I mean, I really love steak."

Doctor: "Sure, that's OK."

Mr. M: "And from time to time, it's OK to have some bacon, right? I mean, there's nothing like bacon sizzling..."

Doctor: "Well, yes, from time to time..."

Mr. M: "And from time to time some ice cream..."

Doctor: "Yes, but..."

Mr. M: "And a hot dog every now and then..."

Doctor: "Well...."

Mr. M: "And some pizza, french fries, and a nice grilled cheese. And now and then a doughnut or two. Deep fried chicken. Of course, the occasional cheeseburger. Every once in a while pasta in a nice cream sauce. A warm cinnamon bun for breakfast, from time to time. Oh, and a cheese omelet! And from time to time..."

Doctor: "Mr. M—excuse me. Other than these foods, from time to time, what else, exactly, do you eat?"

Mr. M: "Ummm...I really can't think of anything."

While any food, in moderation, can be incorporated into a healthful diet, there is a point at which the diet, or overall eating pattern, stops being healthful. And since your eating pattern is made up of the foods you choose, there are indeed foods you should limit. These are the foods that add a lot of what we already have too much of in our diets: saturated fat, trans fat, sugar, cholesterol, and salt, while failing to add the things we could use, such as micronutrients and fiber. An overview of foods to limit to help protect your good eating habits is provided next.

The left column shows a nutrient that should be eaten in limited amount in a healthful diet, and the right column the leading food sources of that nutrient in the typical American diet. By limiting intake of all of the foods in the right column, intake levels of the nutrients listed will be well controlled.

Nutrient	Foods
Saturated Fat*	Meat, including sandwich meats/ hot dogs Whole-fat dairy products: cheese, milk, ice cream, butter, cream Fried foods, fast foods
Trans Fat*	Any product with added "partially hydrogenated oil" Fast food Crackers, chips, popcorn, packaged breads and dessert items Stick margarine
Cholesterol	Egg yolk Meat Organ meats Shrimp & other seafood
Salt	Cheese Chips Deli/luncheon meats/ hot dogs Olives Pickles Pretzels Some packaged breakfast cereals Some packaged soups/stews Tomato juice Instant mashed potatoes Packaged potato, rice, or macaroni entrees Frozen entrees
Sugar	Candy Desserts Sodas/soft drinks Dressings, ketchup Some packaged breakfast cereals Prepackaged sandwich meats Hot dogs

*Restricting intake of total fat, in conjunction with portion control, is also the best means of reducing total calorie intake.

Foods to Prioritize

There are certain foods that are especially helpful in establishing a health-promoting dietary pattern. These are foods that offer a lot of valuable nutrients relative to calories. Other desirable properties of foods include a high satiety index, or tendency to cause a lasting sense of fullness, and a high fiber content. Finally, foods offering essential nutrients that are not widely distributed in the food supply, such as omega-3 fatty acids, are also especially valuable.

This table shows important nutrients or nutrient classes in the left column, and the leading food sources of these nutrients in the right column. These are the nutritional powerhouses that every health-conscious eater should be sure to include in his or her diet.

Nutrient / Nutrient Class	Leading Sources
Antioxidant Vitamins	Brightly colored fruits; brightly colored vegetables; fruit juices; green tea
Calcium	Dairy products, nonfat; green, leafy vegetables (spinach, kale, Swiss chard, broccoli); nuts, almonds
Essential Amino Acids	Beans; egg white; lentils; poultry/fish/meat; soy/tofu
Essential Fatty Acids/ Omega-3 Fatty Acids	Fish, salmon, mackerel, tuna, cod; flaxseed, flaxseed oil; nuts, walnuts; soybeans; seafood, shrimp; wheat germ
Fiber, Insoluble	Wheat bran; whole grains
Fiber, Soluble	Barley; brown rice; fruits, berries, apples; legumes, lentils, chick peas; oats/oat bran; vegetables; carrots
Folate	Beans; green leafy vegetables (spinach, broccoli); oranges; peas; whole grains
Monounsaturated Fatty Acids	Avocados; nuts, walnuts, almonds, cashews, macadamia nuts, peanuts, pecans, hazelnuts, pistachios; olive oil; olives
Overall (Nutrition "super stars")	Broccoli; soybeans; spinach

Glycemic Index: Use & Limitations

The glycemic index indicates how much a food raises blood sugar levels relative to a slice of white bread, which is used as the reference standard. Because insulin is required to move sugar, or glucose, from the blood into cells of the body, when glucose levels rise, insulin levels rise. High insulin levels may contribute to weight gain, and are potentially harmful to blood vessels. For these and other reasons, foods with a high glycemic index are considered potentially harmful to health. In diabetes especially, recommendations tend to focus on the restriction or avoidance of high glycemic index foods.

However, we don't eat just a single food. We eat foods in combinations, over the course of a day, many days, weeks, months, and years. These foods interact with one another in important ways. High-fiber foods tend to lower the blood sugar response to high glycemic index foods, for example. Blood sugar and blood insulin levels will tend to be lower when body weight is lower. So, the ways in which foods influence weight regulation over time (see Resource 9) may matter more in control of blood sugar and insulin levels than the glycemic index per se.

In our view, the glycemic index is worth knowing about, and is of some use in diabetes. Otherwise, we encourage focusing on the overall eating pattern rather than the glycemic index of individual foods as the best way to control weight, blood sugar, and blood insulin.

This table shows and explains the glycemic index of some common foods.

Glycemic Index Use & Limitations

The glycemic index (GI) of some commonly eaten foods is shown. Limitations to the use of the glycemic index as a guide to good eating are shown by the bold entries. Pure sugar and ice cream have a lower glycemic index than white bread, while carrots have a higher glycemic index. Despite this, carrots are a far better choice for good nutrition than sugar, ice cream, or white bread.

Food Group	Food	Glycemic Index
Breads	White bread*	100
	Whole-wheat bread	99
	Pumpernickel	78

(continued)

Food Group	Food	Glycemic Index
		(continued)
Cereal products	White rice	83
	Spaghetti	66
	Barley	31
	Bulgur wheat	65
	Cornflakes	119
	Shredded wheat	97
	Oatmeal	85
Fruit	Bananas	79
	Apples	53
	Oranges	66
	Grapes	62
	Cherries	32
	Raisins	93
Vegetables	Boiled potato	81
	Baked potato	135
	Corn	87
	Peas	74
	Carrots	133
	Yams	74
	Parsnips	141
Legumes	Lima beans	115
	Baked beans	60
	Chick peas	49
	Red lentils	43
	Peanuts	19
Dairy products	Milk	49
	Yogurt	52
	Ice cream	52
Sugar	Sucrose	86

*White bread is the reference standard.

Adapted from: Katz, D.L., *Nutrition in Clinical Practice*. Philadelphia, PA: Lippincott Williams & Wilkins, 2000. Reprinted with permission of the publisher.

Salt & Sodium

- Sodium is one of two minerals in standard table salt, the other being chloride. Sodium is also added to foods in the form of baking soda (sodium bicarbonate), and a variety of flavor enhancers and preservatives.

- The importance of limiting sodium intake is still debated, although the evidence is now clear that sodium in the diet influences blood pressure. Sodium may also affect bone and kidney health. Because of the apparent benefits of limiting sodium intake, and the fact that a health-promoting dietary pattern based largely on unprocessed foods will be naturally low in sodium, we recommend restricting sodium intake to less than 2,400 mg per 2,000 kcal, and ideally, to 1,200 mg per 2,000 kcal.

- Sodium accounts for approximately 40 percent of the weight of salt. The recommendation to limit sodium intake to 2,400 mg/day therefore translates into a salt intake of not more than 6,000 mg (6 grams) per day. This is roughly the amount of salt that would fill up one teaspoon.

- Unlike the preference for sugar, which we are born with, salt is an acquired taste, learned from habit. You can liberate your taste buds from the allure of salt both by acclimating to a lower salt intake in general, and by using the flavors of other spices, juices, and fresh herbs to replace salt. (See Resource 10.)

- Most salt in the diet comes from processed foods, rather than salt you shake on your serving, although both contribute. Eating a diet based largely on natural grains, fruit, and vegetables will result in reduced sodium intake.

- Pickles, olives, capers, and packaged soups, stews, and frozen entrees tend to contain high levels of sodium.

- When salt in a product is visible, such as on hard or soft pretzels, sodium intake can be reduced just by brushing off some of the surface salt.

- In most food categories, there are products that are relatively low in sodium; see Resource 4 for specific product recommendations. Make a particular effort to find low-sodium breads, soups, crackers, chips, spreads, and sauces if trying to reduce your salt intake.

- Make limited use of a salt shaker, and avoid salting food before tasting it.
- What the sodium claims on food labels mean:
  Sodium or salt free: less than 5 mg sodium per serving
  Low sodium: 140 mg sodium or less per serving
  Very low sodium: 35 mg or less per serving
  Reduced sodium: at least 25 percent less sodium than the standard version of the product

Here's a look at what processing does to the sodium content of the following foods:

The Effects of Food Processing on Sodium Content

Natural Food Sodium Content	Processed Food Sodium Content
Baked potato, 8 mg	Potato chips, snack size bag, 600 mg
	Large order of french fries, 350 mg
	Instant mashed potatoes, 770 mg
	Potato *au gratin*, 355 mg
Fresh ear of corn, 15mg	Corn chips, 7 oz bag, 630 mg
	Cornflakes, 230 mg
	Cheese popcorn, 840 mg
Fresh broccoli, 27 mg	Frozen broccoli & cheese sauce, 330 mg
	Canned cream of broccoli soup, 770 mg
Brown rice, 5 mg	Rice and sauce, 900 mg

Soy Facts

- Soy is a very versatile food derived from the soybean. It is extremely popular in Asian cooking, and increasingly popular in Western diets as well.
- Soy takes many forms, from tofu to soy milk, soy nuts, soybeans for cooking, soybean pods (edamame), and soy cheeses, etc.
- The nutritional benefits of soy include an excellent protein profile (i.e., a full complement of amino acids); fiber; essential fatty acids; antioxidants; other micronutrients; and phytoestrogens. Phytoestrogens are nutrients that activate some of the same receptors in the body as the hormone estrogen, potentially conferring benefits to the skeletal and cardiovascular systems.
- Because of its excellent protein content, soy makes a good substitute for meat.
- Many health benefits are attributed to soy, from reducing cancer risk, to controlling symptoms of menopause. Most of these remain under investigation.
- Soy counts among the nutrition powerhouse foods, and is recommended as a regular component of the *way to eat.*

Sugar Substitutes

- Direct, adverse effects of simple sugar on health appear to be limited. Sugar can promote tooth decay, particularly if dental hygiene is not adequate. High sugar intake is of course not desirable in diabetes. But other than these conditions, the adverse effects of sugar are mostly indirect. One of the "indirect" harmful effects of sugar is that it can serve as a vehicle for fat. Many sugary foods also contain saturated or trans fat. The sugar makes them tastier and more appealing, and contributes to excess fat intake.
- The satiety threshold for sugar is high, so appetite remains "turned on" for longer when eating sweet food. Sugar in food often comes along with fat as noted, and

in combination the two are a major contributor to excess calorie intake, and consequently, to weight gain.

- Finally, a health-promoting diet based on natural foods provides limited simple sugar; if the diet is high in simple sugar, it's a clear sign that the overall dietary pattern is not optimal. For these reasons, we support limiting simple sugar intake to less than 10 percent of total calories.
- The best way to limit sugar intake is to eat natural, unprocessed foods. In the context of such an eating pattern, sugar substitutes are an adjunct, or supplemental, means of reducing total sugar consumption.

Sugar Substitutes

Category of Sugar Substitute	Chemical Name	Brand Name
Non-nutritive Intense Sweeteners/Non-bulking	Saccharine	Sweet 'N Low, Sugar Twin Sweet Mate, Sweet 10
	Aspartame*	Equal, NutraSweet
	Acesulfame-K	Sunnet, Sweet One
	Sucralose	Splenda
Bulking Agents	Sorbitol**	
	Xylitol	
	Mannitol	
Natural Alternatives to Sucrose	Fructose**, also called levulose	High-fructose corn syrup (HFCS), Crystalline fructose

*Aspartame contains phenylalanine. Persons with the genetic disorder phenylketonuria (PKU) need to monitor their intake of phenylalanine.

- There are two basic types of sugar substitutes. Intense sweeteners provide sweet taste, but take up almost no space in food; they are particularly used in drinks. Bulking agents add both sweetness and as the name suggests, bulk, and are used in candies, gum, and some baked goods.

Finally, there are natural alternatives to table sugar, or sucrose, often used in processed foods. Some of these influence insulin release differently from sucrose. The following table lists some common sugar substitutes by category, their calorie content, and their effects on blood sugar levels and insulin release. Standard table sugar is made up of sucrose. Sucrose provides 4 kcal per gram.

Calorie Content (kcal/gram)	Use in Baking and Cooking	Effects on Blood Sugar Levels and Insulin Release
0	Yes	None
Negligible	No, may lose sweetness when heated; may add after cooking	None
0	Yes, but won't provide bulk as sugar does	None
0	Yes	None
2	No	None
2	No	None
2	No	None
4	No	May result in slightly less insulin release than sucrose

**Sorbitol and Fructose may have a laxative effect when eaten in large amounts.

Sources: www.diabetes.org; *Sweet Talk: Facts about Sweeteners* from the American Dietetic Association.

Supplement Guide

- Overall, there is far more evidence linking nutrients from foods with health benefits than there is for nutrients in supplement form. No combination of supplements can substitute for a healthful way of eating. This, by the way, is why they are called nutritional "supplements," and not nutritional "substitutes"!

- Efforts to limit calorie intake will reduce the total amount eaten each day, which will tend to reduce intake of micronutrients. For this reason, a multivitamin/mineral supplement is considered reasonable for most adults. Children's vitamins are often reasonable supplements to a healthful eating pattern as well, but it's best to consult your pediatrician for individualized recommendations.

- Fluoride supplements in children's vitamins may be inappropriate if the water in your home is fluoridated. Excessive fluoride intake can mottle children's teeth. Consult your family dentist for individualized guidance.

- The health benefits of omega-3 fatty acids are clear, and most diets in the U.S. are deficient in this vital nutrient class. Unless you eat fish often, or use flaxseeds and/or flaxseed oil regularly, we recommend a flax or fish oil supplement providing one gram of omega-3 fatty acids, twice daily.

- Folate is very valuable to women around the time of conception to prevent a type of birth defect (neural tube defects). The food supply (grains) has been fortified with folate to address this issue, but levels of intake are still sometimes less than optimal. We recommend a prenatal vitamin be started as soon as there is interest in or chance of getting pregnant, rather than after pregnancy is diagnosed. A standard multivitamin with 400 µg of folate is a reasonable alternative prior to pregnancy.

- Antioxidant supplements are popular, but their value is far from certain; a diet rich in antioxidants is of much more clearly established value. Given these considerations, those interested in extra antioxidants should drink green tea, eat plenty of fruits and vegetables, and consider supplements of vitamin E, 200–400IU, in combination with vitamin C, 200–500 mg. The lower end of these dose ranges will be provided by most high-potency multivitamins. We do not specifically recommend antioxidants in supplement form, other than those included in a multivitamin.

- Calcium is generally an important supplement for women in particular. If calcium intake from food is below the recommended level of 1,000 mg to 1,500 mg per day, a supplement is advisable to help keep bones strong. Calcium may also help prevent symptoms of premenstrual syndrome (see Step 9). Calcium can be obtained from nonfat dairy products and fortified foods. If intake is still below the recommended levels, we advise a supplement, such as Tums, providing 500 mg of calcium, taken once or twice each day. To make sure you are getting the calcium you need, discuss use of a supplement with your health-care provider.

- There are many micronutrients used at high doses to prevent, or help manage, diseases and disease risk factors. The selection of such nutrients, their dosing, and assessment of their safety in combination with one another and medication should be addressed with guidance from a knowledgeable health-care professional.

Reasonable Micronutrient Supplements*

- High-potency multivitamin/mineral daily
- Fish or flaxseed oil supplement, 1 gram twice daily
- Calcium supplement (women especially), 500 mg once or twice daily
- Additional single nutrient supplements for specific health benefits only with expert advice (health-care professional and/or dietitian)

*Tailored guidance from a health-care professional regarding use of supplements is advisable.

Resource 3: The Way to Evaluate Your Diet

As discussed in Step 1, adopting a health-promoting dietary pattern requires a candid assessment of your actual diet. The materials provided and referenced here give you the means to make an accurate, detailed, and enlightening assessment of your usual eating habits.

Your Diet Diary

Use the following food diary to conduct an initial assessment of your eating habits, as discussed in Step 1.

Food Diary Chart

Meal/snack	Descriptors	Day of the week	Date	Work day? Y / N
Pre-breakfast	What			
	How much			
	When			
	Where			
	Why			
Breakfast	What			
	How much			
	When			
	Where			
	Why			
A.M. Snack(s)	What			
	How much			
	When			
	Where			
	Why			

Meal/snack	Descriptors	Day of the week	Date	Work day? Y / N
Lunch	What			
	How much			
	When			
	Where			
	Why			
P.M. Snack(s)	What			
	How much			
	When			
	Where			
	Why			
Dinner	What			
	How much			
	When			
	Where			
	Why			
Evening Snack(s)	What			
	How much			
	When			
	Where			
	Why			
Other (e.g., alcohol, gum, etc.)	What			
	How much			
	When			
	Where			
	Why			

Print Resources for Assessing the Nutritional Composition of Foods

The following are full-length books that provide a detailed nutrient composition of thousands of commonly eaten foods, along with tips and guidance for analyzing your diet:

Margen, Sheldon, et al. (eds). *The Wellness Nutrition Counter.* New York, NY: HealthLetter Associates, 1997.

Morrill, Judi S., Bakun, Sheri, Murphy, Suzanne P., *Are You Eating Right?* Menlo Park, CA: Orange Grove Publishing, 1997.

Online/Software Resources for Assessing the Nutritional Composition of Foods

As those of you who use the Internet know, websites tend to come and go. Those listed below are current as of the printing of this book. However, if these fail to meet your needs, or if you find they are not functioning when you log on, select your preferred Internet search engine and enter the term "dietary intake analysis" to find a list of websites providing this service. In general, those sites sponsored by professional organizations, universities, or the government are the most reliable; avoid sites that are promoting any particular product.

The nutritional composition of most foods can be obtained by using the USDA's nutrient database for standard reference:

http://www.nal.usda.gov/fnic/cgi-bin/nut_search.pl

The Nutrition Analysis Tool is available free online through a website sponsored by the Food Science and Human Nutrition Department at the University of Illinois: http://www.nat.uiuc.edu/

The home page for Foodcount.com, a service that provides access to nutrition analysis software and related materials online for an annual fee:

http://www.foodcount.com/Index.cfm?Method=Home

A website particularly devoted to analyzing the nutritional composition of fast food: http://www.fatcalories.com/

A free site that allows for assessment of both diet and activity level: http://www.fitday.com/

Click on "Nutrition Calculator" and enter your food diary items for a free personalized nutritional analysis:

www.dietwatch.com

Provides a free personalized nutritional analysis and much more. A well-organized and comprehensive website for anyone interested in being well-informed about nutrition, health, and fitness:
www.webdietitian.com
Other sites of potential use and interest:
http://www.dietsure.com/
http://www.healthy.net/AANP/Bookstore/N2DietSoft.html
http://www.nuconnexions.com/DietAnalysis/
http://www.eDiets.com

Common Food Generalizations

As discussed in Step 1, many of us have the tendency to think that foods that can be called by the same name must have the same nutritional value. But of course, they don't. There are a number of food "categories" that are subject to very wide variation in nutrient composition. So, pay close attention to the actual foods you eat in these categories, because they are not at all the same.

Food Category	What to Look Out For
Bread	Added oils; use of spreads
Breakfast items, such as pancakes	Wide variety in the fat and calorie content; addition of condiments such as butter, amount of added syrup, whether natural or artificial
Cereal	Added sugar, salt, and oil; low fiber content
Chicken, turkey	Method of cooking (frying adds fat and calories); dark vs. white meat (white meat is leaner); with or without skin (skin adds fat and calories)
Chips/crackers/ popcorn (especially pre-popped kind)	Added fat; salt
Many categories of baked goods, such as muffins, coffees cakes, etc.	Wide variety in the fat, sugar, and calorie content

Food Category	What to Look Out For	(continued)
Pasta	High-fat sauces; egg noodles	
Pizza	Amount of added cheese; pepperoni, sausage, dough with added fat; tomato sauce with added fat	
Salad	Addition of croutons, cheese, or meat; use of iceberg lettuce rather than more nutritious varieties; type of dressing	
Salad dressing	Creamy dressings; bleu cheese dressing	
Sandwiches	Use of high-fat spreads such as mayonnaise, butter, or margarine; addition of cheese slices; fatty meats; white bread	
Soup	Added fat; salt	

Foods Commonly Overlooked

Some foods are so easy to munch or gulp that you may not even realize you're eating them! These are the foods that add calories, fat, salt, and/or sugar to our diets that we tend to overlook.

Note to Moms and Dads: Be careful about finishing the scraps of food your kids leave on their plates—these calories count, too!

Note to Cooks: Be careful about the tasting and nibbling that can go on while preparing food.

Bear in mind that this list is not comprehensive. Your diet will have its own particular "stow-away" foods, and it may take a pretty thorough inspection to find them all!

Food	What It Adds to Your Diet
Alcoholic beverages	Calories
Candies, gum	Sugar, fat, calories
Cheese slices	Fat, calories
Chips/crackers/popcorn	Fat, salt, calories
Condiments such as croutons, bacon bits, etc.	Fat, calories, salt
Cream and sugar in coffee	Fat, sugar, calories
Dressings on salads	Fat, calories
Grated cheese	Fat, calories
Nuts, such as pistachios	Fat, calories; often salt
Sauces on entrees	Fat, calories; often salt
Seeds, such as sunflower seeds	Fat, calories; often salt
Soft drinks, soda	Sugar, calories
Spreads (mayonnaise, margarine, butter, cream cheese)	Fat, calories
Unplanned eating, such as foods brought by others to work	Fat, sugar, calories

Leading Sources of Fat, Sugar, & Calories in the Typical American Diet

Our modern diets tend to have far too much sugar, salt, and total fat, especially saturated and trans fat. These can be reduced substantially by focusing on the relatively short list of major sources, as shown below.

Reduce the Following	By Cutting Back on These Leading Sources
Calories	Fatty meats; deli meats; cheese and other dairy products; fast food/fried food; chips; nuts; sweets; sodas; beer
Sodium	Packaged soups, stews; packaged potatoes (instant mashed, scalloped, *au gratin*, etc.) and pasta or rice (with cheese sauce); deli meats; olives; pickles; snack foods such as chips and pretzels; canned goods, cheeses
Saturated fat	Fatty meats; deli meats; cheese and other dairy products including whole-fat milk, butter; fast food/fried food; banana chips
Sugar	Sweets; soda and other soft drinks; highly processed breakfast cereals and baked goods; ketchup, some mustards
Trans fat	Fried foods; stick margarine; processed food of many varieties; non-dairy creamer

Resource 4: The Way to Shop

The food available to you in your home determines the safety of your personal nutritional environment. Food at home begins with what makes it into your shopping cart. The entries here provide the necessary details for skillful, thoughtful, healthful shopping.

Basic Shopping Skills

- Don't shop when hungry. This often results in impulsive purchases. Have a nutritious snack or meal before shopping, and base your selection on your knowledge of good nutrition, rather than a transient craving.
- Use a shopping list that helps you stick with your "plan" for bringing home healthful foods.
- Read the food and ingredient labels of any new or unfamiliar product and assess the content of calories, fat, types of fat, salt, sugar, and fiber.
- Get to know preferred brands and products so you can make your healthful purchases at a glance.
- Take advantage of the layout of a supermarket for some physical activity; even if your purchases are limited to an aisle or two, walk all of the aisles and perimeter of the store.
- Look for a "natural" or "health" food section to shop for: cereals, chips, mixes, soups, dips, and spreads.
- For food safety, make your selections from the store perimeter, where refrigerated items are kept, last, so they don't warm up in your cart as you go up and down the aisles.

Interpretation of Food Labels

- Reading food labels isn't necessarily fun. But it is very important, rewarding, and with a little guidance, pretty straightforward. By reading labels, you take control of your eating habits, and those of your family, into your own hands—and out of those of the advertising executives who design product packages to catch your eye!

Fat, All Fat, and Nothing but Fat...

Consider a tablespoon of oil. It has roughly 126 calories, and 14 grams of fat.

All of the calories are from fat:

Calories = 126   Fat calories = 126

So, if you calculate the percent calories from fat, you get:

(126 / 126) X 100 = 100%

But the %DV is the portion of all fat calories in a day you get from that tablespoon of oil. If you eat 2,000 kcal a day, and 30 percent of those comes from fat, you eat 600 fat calories, or 67 grams of fat, per day.

The % DV for fat in the tablespoon of oil is:

(126 / 600) X 100 = 21%

This doesn't change the fact that the oil is all fat! So, to track fat without using a computer, just consider the percent of calories in the serving that come from fat. If you eat plenty of grains, vegetables, and fruit, and select packaged foods that generally have less than 30 percent of calories from fat, your diet will wind up being relatively low in fat.

Who do you think cares more about your health, or that of your family?

- What a food really is, and the effects it has on your health, depend not on what it's called, but on the ingredients and nutrients it actually contains. Use food labels to make nutritious choices, and then just stick with them; you only need to read the label when selecting a new product, or when an old product changes. If you "are what you eat," then it is best to know exactly what that is! By focusing on just a few key figures on a nutrition label, you will be able to decide if that particular food item fits in well with your way to eat.

A "Tip" about Food Labels and Fat...

It's pretty customary to leave a tip when you eat out at a restaurant, usually 15–20 percent. This custom comes in handy for calculating the percent of fat calories in a serving!

Think of the total calories in the serving as you would the price of the meal. Using 20 percent (go on, be generous!), calculate the amount you would leave as a tip. If the fat calories are less than the tip amount, it's a low-fat food. If just slightly over the tip amount, it's a food with relatively low to moderate fat content. And if there is much more fat calories in the serving then there are dollars in your tip, then you may want to take this tip instead: eat something else!

Of course, even a relatively low-fat diet can, and should, accommodate some foods high in fat; but it won't remain a relatively low-fat diet for long if too many of your food choices are high in fat!

- In general, your goal should be to choose packaged foods that are low in fat, low in sodium, and high in fiber, and to eat them in reasonable amounts!
  1. Check the serving size. Use the serving size as a guide to your own portions. Remember, portion control is key to maintaining a life-long healthy weight.
  2. Look at the number of total fat grams. Use a simple rule of 3:3 grams of fat or less per serving is generally a relatively low-fat food. This rule is not so useful if the serving size is much less than 100 calories. If you don't mind a little more math, follow this formula:

(Fat calories / Total calories) X 100 = percent of calories from fat

     If that number is less than 30 percent, it's a relatively low-fat food. If that number is less than 20 percent, it's a low-fat food.
- Bear in mind that food labels do not tell you the percent of calories from fat in a product. They tell you the percent

of the recommended total daily fat intake ("percent Daily Value," or "%DV") found in a serving of the product. Why? Probably because the "percent daily value" is a much smaller number, and therefore generally sounds better! But it can be rather misleading, as shown on the next page.

3. Evaluate the amount of sodium. Here use the reference number of 2,400 mg, the total amount of sodium milligrams recommended per day. How much of the allotted 2,400 mg does this product use? You can also think about the ratio of sodium to calories. To keep your sodium intake at or below the recommended 2,400 mg per day in a 2,000 kcal diet requires that you not take in more than about 1.2 mg of sodium per calorie. So any food that provides more than 120 mg of sodium per 100 kcal can be considered a "relatively high sodium food." If you eat few high sodium foods, and plenty of low sodium foods, your overall diet will be naturally low in sodium.

4. Look at the number of grams of fiber. If fiber isn't listed, there is none! Again apply the rule of 3:3 grams or more of fiber per serving is a fiber-rich food. Look for breads and cereals with at least 2 grams of fiber, and preferably 3 or more, per 100 kcal.

5. Where do you find out if there is any trans fat in the product? Depending on your visual acuity, and the size of the package, you may need your magnifying glass, because the information is pretty well hidden at times! Look on the Ingredient List for the term partially hydrogenated before the name of different types of oils. Usually you'll find "partially hydrogenated soybean and/or cottonseed oil." Ingredients are listed in order of quantity, with the most abundant items listed first. So try to avoid products with added partially hydrogenated oils, but especially avoid those that list such oils within the first three or so ingredients.

The Food Label, Demystified

Example: *Cape Cod Reduced Fat Potato Chips*

Nutrition Facts

Serving size 1 oz. (28g/about 19 chips)
Servings per container 5

Amount per serving

Calorie 130   Calories from Fat 50

	% Daily Value
Total Fat 6g	**9%**
Saturated Fat 2g	3%
Polyunsaturated Fat 2g	
Monounsaturated Fat 3.5g	
Cholesterol 0mg	**0%**
Sodium 110mg	**5%**
Total Carbohydrate 18g	**6%**
Dietary Fiber 1g	4%
Sugars Less than 1g	
Protein 2g	

Vitamin A 0%	•	Vitamin C 10%
Calcium 0%	•	Iron 2%

• Percent Daily Values (DV) are based on a 2,000 calorie diet. Your daily values may be higher or lower depending on your calorie needs:

	Calories	2,000	2,500
Total Fat	Less than	65g	80g
Sat Fat	Less than	20g	25g
Cholesterol	Less than	300mg	300mg
Sodium	Less than	2,400mg	2,400mg
Total Carbohydrate		300g	375g
Dietary Fiber		25g	30g

Calories per gram:
Fat 9 • Carbohydrate 4 • Protein 4

The fat content has been reduced from 10 grams for regular potato chips to 6 grams per serving.

INGREDIENTS: Potatoes, Canola Oil, and Salt

The total calories from fat per serving: a priority! Divide this by the calories per serving, then multiply by 100 to get the % calories from fat. [(50/130)X100]=38%. So, this is a fat-reduced product, but NOT a low-fat product.

This is the percent of total recommended fat intake for the day, assuming a 2,000 kcal diet, provided in a serving. In this case, it's 6 grams of fat, divided by 65 grams, and multiplied by 100: [(6/65)X100]=9%. Note that this can make it seem as if a product is lower in fat than is actually is.

This is simply the total calories in ONE serving. Note that serving sizes vary. If the serving size is approximately 100 kcal, apply the "**1,2,3 rule.**"*

The fiber per serving; prioritize products with at least 2, and preferably 3 grams of fiber per 100 kcal serving.

When included, this box shows recommended intakes for an entire day using current U.S.DA guidelines.

A description of how this product was reduced in fat relative to the standard product.

Ingredients are listed separately from the nutrient facts. In general, prioritize foods with a short list of natural ingredients. Recall that ingredients are listed in order of quantity; the first items are most abundant.

***1,2,3 Rule:** look for products that provide for every **100 calories** at least **2** grams of **fiber** and not more than **3** grams of **fat**, and you will be cruising right along the *way to eat!*

What the Food Label Meant to Say...

Regarding Fat...

What the Label Says	What the Label Means
Fat Free	Less than 0.5 gram fat
Low Fat	3 grams of fat or less
Reduced Fat	At least 25% less fat than the standard product
Cholesterol Free	Less than 2 mg cholesterol and 2 g or less of saturated fat
Low Cholesterol	20 mg or less cholesterol and 2 g or less saturated fat
Reduced Cholesterol	At least 25% less cholesterol than the standard product, and 2 g or less saturated fat

Regarding Sodium...

What the Label Says	What the Label Means
Sodium Free	Less than 5 mg sodium
Very Low Sodium	35 mg or less sodium
Low Sodium	140 mg or less sodium
Reduced Sodium	At least 25% less sodium than the standard product
Light in Sodium	50% less sodium than the standard product

Regarding Calories...

What the Label Says	What the Label Means
Calorie Free	Less than 5 calories
Low Calorie	40 calories or less

Between the Lines...

- Beware of the "baked" labels on crackers and chips. Although it generally means that the product is lower in fat than its standard counterpart, the percentage of calories from fat is often still well above the recommended upper limit of 30 percent, and there is often partially hydrogenated oil (trans fat) as part of the mix. You can certainly include these foods in a healthful diet, but you cannot count on them to pull your fat intake down!
- If a product is labeled "reduced fat," you can generally be sure it's not low in fat, or it would say so! Reduced fat products are often still high in fat, just lower than the standard version of the particular product.

Interpreting a food label is not all that tough, but you also have to know how to read between the lines!

Light or Lite	1/3 fewer calories or 50% less fat than the standard product; if more than half the calories are from fat, fat content must be reduced by 50% or more

Regarding Sugar...

What the Label Says	What the Label Means
Sugar Free	Less than 0.5 g sugar
Reduced Sugar	At least 25% less sugar than the standard product

Source: Browne, Mona Boyd, *Label Facts for Healthful Eating*. Chicago, IL: American Dietetic Association, 1993.

Recommended Brands & Products
A "Virtual" Trip to the Supermarket

This table shows the category or food group in the left column and recommended varieties, products, product lines, or brands in the right column. When a brand name is listed alone, the entire product line is recommended. When a food is described but no brand name is provided, any product matching the description is recommended. You may not find each of these brands of products in the grocery store you use. Look for others with high nutritional standards—there are many more.

Food Category	Recommended Products & Brands
Baking Goods	
Flour	Arrowhead Mills; whole-grain flours
Other	All natural vanilla; bittersweet or semi-sweet chocolate, Ghirardelli double-chocolate chocolate chips
Beverages	
Juice	Natural 100% juices without added sugar; orange juice with added calcium
Bottled Water	Naturally flavored mineral water; sparkling water
Tea	Green tea, herbal teas; Honest T; iced teas without added sugar
Coffee creamer	Use undiluted nonfat powdered milk (e.g., Carnation); avoid other creamers
Cocoa	Ovaltine Chocolate Malt; fat-free varieties of chocolate milk and hot cocoa
Soda	Choose diet sodas; restricted intake of all brands is recommended
Breads & Baked Goods	
Breads	Whole-grain breads without added oils; The Baker product line; Vermont Bread Company; Alvarado St. Bakery; Joseph's Lavash roll-ups, whole

Food Category	Recommended Products & Brands *(continued)*
	wheat; select varieties with at least 2 grams of fiber and less than 3 grams of fat per 100 calorie serving; avoid products with partially hydrogenated oils
Rolls	Whole-grain rolls; avoid added fat; select varieties with 1 or more grams of fiber and less than 3 grams of fat per 100 calorie serving
Muffins	Most muffins are high in fat and calories and should be restricted or avoided; choose nonfat or low-fat muffins; Thomas' English Muffins, oat bran and honey wheat

Breakfast Entrees

Waffles, Pancakes	Van's waffles; avoid toaster pastries

Cereals

Cold	Nature's Path; Kashi; Lifestream; Barbara's; Health Valley; Arrowhead Mills; Post Raisin Bran; Post Shredded Wheat 'N Bran; Post Grapenuts; Kellogg's Complete; General Mills Cheerios; General Mills Fiber One; General Mills Oatmeal Crisps; General Mills Multi-Bran Chex; Quaker Life; Quaker Toasted Oatmeal Squares; Grainfield's; Kretschmer Wheat Germ; New Morning
Hot	Quaker Oats; Mother's 100% Multigrain; Hodgson Mill; Kashi; other whole-grain varieties (look for at least 2 grams of fiber per serving); John McCann's Irish Oatmeal

Cookies

	Barbara's; Frookie; Health Valley; Barry's Bakery; Look for 3 grams or less of fat per serving and avoid products with partially hydrogenated oils.

Crackers/Pretzels

	Wasa; Kavli; FinnCrisp; Ryvita; Health Valley; Ak-Mak

Food Category	Recommended Products & Brands *(continued)*
Dairy Products	
Milk	Skim (fat-free milk); Skim Plus; Simply Smart; Soy-milk and low-fat soy-milk as a nondairy alternative
Cheese	Limit types with 8 grams or more of fat per ounce. Look for low-fat, part-skim, or nonfat varieties including ricotta, part-skim mozzarella, string, feta, goat, and Neufchâtel. Use freshly grated Parmesan.
Cottage cheese	Fat-free cottage cheese
Yogurt	Fat-free varieties with active cultures; Dannon Danimals low-fat drinkable yogurt; Stonyfield Farm organic Yosqueeze portable yogurt (especially for kids)
Deli	Avoid processed meats and salads with added mayonnaise; skinless, oven-roasted turkey breast is a preferred item
Desserts	Look for fat-free or fat-reduced varieties; see cookies, frozen foods
Dips & Salsa	
Dips	Hummus; guacamole; taboule; black bean dip
Salsa	Fresh salsa (produce section); choose from many varieties without added oil
Dressings	
Salad dressings	Cain's; vinaigrettes; no-oil dressings; avoid cream and cheese based varieties; avoid low-fat varieties with added sugar; use olive oil and balsamic vinegar
Other	Marinades and chutneys without added fat/oil

Food Category	Recommended Products & Brands _(continued)_
Canned Goods/Dried Goods	
Cooking grains	Wild rice; brown rice; couscous; bulgur wheat; pearled barley; wheat berries; kashi
Canned Chili	Health Valley; Fantastic dry vegetarian chili mix
Canned fish	Canned salmon in water; canned mackerel in water; Starkist Albacore Tuna in water (no-drain package for convenience)
Beans	Goya (many varieties; choose assorted colors); vegetarian baked beans; dried fava beans; dried soy beans; dried flageolet beans; dry canneli beans
Legumes	Chick peas (garbanzo beans); red lentils; green lentils; French lentils (brown); soybeans; split peas
Dried fruit	Raisins; currants; figs; dates; apricots; peaches; pears; dried whole bananas (avoid the banana chips); choose varieties without added sugar
Eggs	Omega-3 fatty acid enriched eggs
Ethnic	
Asian	Lite soy sauce; lite teriyaki sauce
Spanish	Goya Recaito, Sofrito, and Sazon seasonings
Tex-Mex	Soft fat-free or low-fat tortillas; Old El Paso nonfat refried beans; bean dips
Frozen Foods	
Frozen entrees	Gardenburger; Boca Burgers; Lean Cuisine; Weight Watchers Smart Ones; Healthy Choice
Frozen desserts	Sorbet (not sherbet); nonfat frozen yogurt; fruit juice bars; Good Humor Fat-free Fudgsicles
Frozen fruits	Assorted berries, cantaloupe balls packed without added sugar
Frozen vegetables	Select a "rainbow" of colors; look for products packed plain without added sauces

Food Category	Recommended Products & Brands *(continued)*
Meat	Fresh fish; fresh or frozen shrimp; skinless poultry (white meat); loin and round cuts of meat with visible fat trimmed
Mixes	
Dessert mixes	Angel food cake mix
Pancake mix	Arrowhead Mills Maple Grove Farms of Vermont
Quick breads & muffins	Hodgson Mill
Entrees	Near East falafel; Fantastic Vegetarian Burger; Fantastic Tofu Burger; Fantastic product line
Oils	Olive oil extra virgin (first cold pressed is best); canola oil; Barlean's flaxseed oil (cold use only)
Pasta	Semolina pasta; whole-wheat pasta; avoid egg noodles
Preserves, Honey, Syrup	
Preserves	St. Dalfour; Fiordifrutta; Sorrell Ridge; Polaner All Fruit; Hero
Honey	Pure natural honeys
Syrup	100% maple syrup
Produce: Fruit	Select a rainbow of colors; fresh fruits in season: blueberries, strawberries, oranges, bananas, mango, kiwi, grapefruit, star fruit, apples, pineapple, all grapes, all melons, etc.
Produce: Vegetables	
Lettuce	Mixed greens; baby spinach; romaine; escarole; prewashed and packaged lettuces for convenience; avoid iceberg
Other	A variety of fresh vegetables in a rainbow of colors; potatoes, tomatoes, onions, cabbage, beans, all varieties of squash, broccoli, peas,

Food Category	Recommended Products & Brands *(continued)*
	carrots, kale, spinach, bell peppers, Brussels sprouts, zucchini, etc.
Produce: Flavor Enhancers	Garlic, ginger root, onions, shallots, mushrooms, tomatillos, fresh salsa, lemons, limes, fresh chives, cilantro, basil
Sauces	
Pasta sauces	Classico Basil & Tomato; Aunt Millie's
Asian	Lite soy sauce; lite teriyaki sauce
Snack Foods: Salty	
Chips	Guiltless Gourmet Baked Chips (many varieties); Frito Lay Baked Tostitos; avoid chips with added hydrogenated oils
Popcorn	Air-popped popcorn; microwave popcorn with limited added oil; Orville Reddenbacher's; PopSecret; avoid prepopped cheese popcorn
Rice Cakes	Any variety made from whole grain rice, without added fat
Nuts / Seeds	Genisoy soy nuts; flaxseeds, dry roasted almonds, peanuts or sunflower seeds without added oil; Planter's Dry Roasted Peanuts, Lightly Salted; Blue Diamond Dry Roasted Almonds
Pretzels	Snyder's of Hanover sourdough, whole-wheat, or oat bran pretzels; other brands with no added fat
Snack Foods: Sweet	
Granola bars / cereal bars	Health Valley; Genisoy
Canned fruit	Fruit in fruit juices (avoid heavy syrup); Del Monte; Dole; Mott's
Pudding	Jell-O Fat-free Pudding Snacks
Apple sauce	Apple sauce without added sugar

Food Category	Recommended Products & Brands *(continued)*
Soup & Stew	
Broth	Swanson's Fat-free Chicken Broth
Soup	Health Valley; Fantastic; The Spice Hunter; Campbell's Healthy Request product line
Spices & Condiments	
Condiments	Olives; capers; artichoke hearts
Spices	Various dried spices and fresh herbs, per taste
Spreads	
Margarine	Smart Balance; Benecol; tub margarines; minimize use, avoid stick margarines
Cream cheese	Nonfat or low-fat varieties are preferred; restrict or avoid
Butter	Avoid, or strictly limit
Mayonnaise	Nonfat or low-fat varieties preferred; restrict or avoid
Nut butters	Almond butter; peanut butter made from peanuts only (e.g., Smucker's Natural Creamy Peanut Butter; Teddie unsalted peanut butter)
Mustard	Gulden's; Grey Poupon
Ketchup	Look for varieties with reduced sugar or salt
Vinegars	Balsamic (highly flavorful); other varieties to suit taste

Resource 5: The Way to Stock Your Pantry

Your ability to provide yourself and/or your family with health-promoting meals and snacks depends on the convenient availability of healthful food choices at home. A well-stocked pantry is the key. These entries offer all of the necessary guidance for the foods, goods, and ingredients one should have in the house to make healthful cooking, and eating, easy and convenient. The pantry is also intended to create a safe nutritional environment in the home, so that the adverse influences and temptations of the prevailing nutritional environment are controlled.

The Way to Eat Pantry: An Overview

Home is probably the place where your choices for eating and food preparation will most often be made. Making your home a safe nutritional environment is therefore a key component of the way to eat. A pantry stocked with nutritious foods puts all you need for healthful cooking, baking, and snacking at your fingertips.

If the *way to eat* is a significant redirect for you, you may want to clear out of your refrigerator, freezer, and cupboards the holdovers from your prior dietary pattern. Then use this guide to stock your pantry. Make the healthful way of eating the path of least resistance, by having nutritious and delicious options for snacks, sandwiches, desserts, and dinners within easy reach, all the time. Open your pantry, and twenty minutes later you'll have a delicious, healthful, convenient meal. A well-stocked pantry is the ultimate in "fast food"—quick, convenient, delicious, and nutritious!

The Well-Stocked Pantry

Dry Grains and Beans

- couscous
- wheat berries
- kashi
- bulgur wheat
- barley
- lentils
- soy beans
- flageolet beans
- small white beans
- baby fava beans
- brown rice
- wild rice
- falafel mix
- veggie burger mix (Fantastic)
- chili mix (Fantastic)
- tofu veggie mix (Fantastic)

- whole-grain bread
- whole-grain bread wraps
- whole-wheat pita

- semolina pasta
  (all shapes and sizes)

Refrigerator Items

- skim milk
- fat-free buttermilk
- orange juice
- other 100 percent fruit juice
- flaxseed oil
- fresh parmesan or romano cheese
- mozzarella cheese, part-skim
- low-fat string cheese
- omega-3 eggs
- fat-free plain yogurt
- nonfat ricotta
- fat-free puddings
- low-fat drinkable yogurts
- tofu
- Dijon mustard
- grainy mustard
- fat-free salsa
- hummus
- avocado
- unsalted peanut butter
- apple butter
- margarine (such as Smart Balance)

- all-fruit preserves
- lemons/limes
- tomatoes
- scallions
- bagged baby carrots
- bagged spinach
- lettuce or bagged mixed greens
- other fresh produce, enough to stay fresh (zucchini, squash, string beans, broccoli, etc.)
- sun-dried tomatoes
- fresh herbs (one bunch at a time to keep fresh—cilantro or parsley or basil or chives)
- roasted red peppers in vinegar (jar)
- horseradish
- olives
- capers
- fat-free polenta
- whole-grain sliced bread

Freezer Items

- frozen strawberries
- frozen blueberries
- lean ground turkey
- filet of sole
- peas

- boneless, skinless chicken and turkey breasts
- shrimp
- salmon steaks or filets
- veggie burgers

- fat-free frozen yogurt
- sorbet
- frozen, baked soft pretzels

- orange juice concentrate
- apple juice concentrate

Canned Products

- chick peas (garbanzos)
- cannellini beans
- black beans
- red kidney beans
- crushed tomatoes
- whole plum tomatoes
- diced tomatoes
- tomato paste

- corn kennels
- canned tuna in water
- canned salmon in water
- canned fat-free refried beans
- canned pumpkin
- canned evaporated skim milk

Seasonings

- garlic powder (not salt)
- nutmeg
- oregano
- paprika
- red pepper flakes
- salt
- thyme leaves
- ground turmeric
- rosemary
- basil
- cinnamon
- coriander
- cumin
- curry

- cilantro
- fennel seeds
- bread crumbs (unsalted)
- cooking wines (vermouth, sherry, red)
- dried mushrooms
- fat-free, low-sodium vegetable broth
- fat-free, low-sodium chicken broth
- low-sodium soy sauce
- fresh black peppercorns and pepper mill

Root Vegetables, Flavor Enhancers

- potatoes (baking, red, yukan gold, sweet, yams)
- fresh garlic
- onions (yellow and red)

- shallots
- fresh ginger root
- fresh garlic cloves

Baking Goods

- flour (whole wheat, white, oat, etc.)
- yeast
- gluten
- cornmeal
- flaxseed meal
- oats
- unsweetened Dutch process cocoa
- brown sugar
- confectioner's sugar
- granulated sugar
- baking powder
- baking soda
- pure vanilla extract
- pure orange extract
- bittersweet chocolate
- semi-sweet chocolate chips

Snack Items

- fresh fruit
- variety of dried fruit:
- raisins
- dates (whole and chopped)
- figs
- apricots
- whole bananas
- pears
- peach
- whole-grain crackers (fat free)
- fat-free pretzels
- fat-free corn chips
- fat-free salsa
- low-fat microwave popcorn
- rice cakes
- homemade trail mix (see Resource 7)
- homemade granola power bars (see recipes, Resource 11)

Breakfast Items

- variety of low-fat dry cereals (see the table in Resource 4 for recommendations)
- muesli
- low-fat granola
- kashi
- steel cut oats
- oatmeal
- pancake mix fresh fruit
- 100 percent maple syrup
- honey

Oils and Vinegars

- canola oil
- olive oil
- flaxseed oil (must be refrigerated)
- balsamic vinegar
- red wine vinegar
- apple cider vinegar

Seeds and Nuts

- sunflower
- pumpkin seeds
- flaxseeds
- pine nuts (pignoli)

- walnuts
- hazelnuts
- almonds
- soy nuts

Priority Food Items for a Safe Nutritional Environment in Your Home

Here are lists to help you make the right decisions: categories of eating in the left column, foods to keep at home for healthful eating in the middle column, and the foods to avoid in the right column.

For Nutritious	Be Sure to Have	And Avoid
Breakfasts	Whole-grain breads	Sugary, low-fiber cereals; Cereals with added fats
	Whole-grain cereals	
	Skim milk	Whole milk; cream / nondairy creamers
	All-fruit preserves	
	Fresh fruit	Bacon, sausage
	100% fruit juice	Toaster pastries or breakfast bars
	Nutritious pancake mix	Muffins
	Nonfat powdered milk	
Lunches	Whole-grain breads	Deli meats
	Nutritious soups or stews	Mayonnaise
		White bread
	Tuna packed in water	Butter
	Sliced turkey breast	Cheese
	Bean salads	
	Fresh fruit	
	Fresh vegetables (e.g., lettuce, tomato, baby carrots)	

For Nutritious	Be Sure to Have	And Avoid	(continued)
Dinners	Cooking grains	Chopped meat	
	Assorted vegetables	Fatty meats	
	Fresh or frozen fish	Cream sauces	
	Skinless poultry		
	Beans		
	Lentils		
Salty Snacks	Baked corn chips	Fried chips	
	Baked potato chips	Nuts with added oil	
	Whole-grain crackers	Crackers with added oil	
	Dry roasted nuts and seeds		
	Baked pretzels		
Sweet Snacks	Fresh fruit	Candy bars	
	Dried fruit	High-fat granola bars	
	Low-fat granola bars	Puddings	
	Trail mix	Muffins	
Desserts	Sorbet	High-fat cakes, cookies	
	Nonfat frozen yogurt	Ice cream	
	Fruit cookies		
Beverages	Water	Soda	
	Skim milk	Juice drinks/cocktails with added sugar	
	100% fruit juice	Whole milk	
	Green tea		
	Mineral water		

Resource 6: The Way to Snack

Many of the strategies offered in Steps 3–6 include a recommendation to snack on health-promoting foods. Advantages of doing so include: avoiding excessive hunger; avoiding fear of hunger; reducing appetite that leads to binges; relieving stress and tension; and shifting the diet to more healthful choices. For snacking to be beneficial, however, the snacks themselves must be well chosen, and used in substitution for, rather than in addition to, other items in the diet. Provided below are categories of healthful snacks, specific food items in each category, suggestions for making the snacks readily available each day and for keeping them fresh and handy, tips on timing, and some suggestions on what these snacks should be replacing in your diet.

Health-promoting Snacks

To get the many advantages that snacking can provide to your overall diet and health, you must choose good snacks. Characteristics of good snacks, and good snacking, are as follows.

- Snacks should be eaten instead of, rather than in addition to, food formerly eaten at meal times. Even the most healthful snacking will lead to weight gain if it is in addition to everything that was eaten before.
- Snacks should be nutrient dense and energy dilute. This means they should provide a lot of vitamins, minerals, and/or fiber in relation to calories. Good snacks don't need to be low-calorie foods, per se, as long as the calories are "worth it" in terms of nutritional value.
- Snacks that are relatively high in calories are good choices only when they are very nutritious, satisfying, and filling. Such snacks are especially helpful in reducing eating at other times, and so make up for the calories they provide.
- Snacks should be quick and convenient to prepare.
- Snacks should be easy to pack up and carry.
- Snacks should generally be easy to eat on the go or at your desk.
- Good snacking should have a certain rhythm, with certain types of snacks eaten at certain times of day. Just as

breakfast foods differ from dinner foods, morning snacks should differ from afternoon snacks. This pattern can of course be modified as you see fit, but some consistency will make choosing easier, will help avoid excessive variety, and will facilitate portion control. Recommended for A.M. snacking are fruit, dried fruit, whole-grain breads, nonfat yogurt, and cereals. P.M. snacking can be based on these same foods, but if not, recommendations are vegetables, dips, whole-grain crackers, and baked chips.

- Good snacking involves good timing. Snacks should be eaten when hungry, and used to reduce calories at mealtime.

- Good snacking should address needs other than hunger. For example, if you are tense or stressed, chewing on something can provide relief along with pleasure. Dried figs, pears or peaches, or dense bread make good choices. If more inclined for something to crunch on, baby carrots, or Shredded Wheat cereal, for example, make good choices.

- Be attentive to the reasons for your snacking. If out of hunger, it may be important to eat something substantial and satisfying. But if, for example, out of boredom, it may be especially important to eat something low in calories. The best low-calorie snacks are fresh vegetables. No one we know has gained weight eating baby carrots; they make a great snack.

- Good snacks combine well with other snack foods. Good combinations include nonfat yogurt, fruit, and cereal; whole-grain bread and dried fruit; vegetables or baked chips and a dip such as humus.

Recommendations for Healthful Snacking

Fresh fruit. Almost any fresh fruit in season is a good choice. Apples, bananas, oranges, grapes, cherries, pears, peaches, nectarines, tangerines, clementines, melon, and berries are great. Fruits that are convenient to eat, such as apples, grapes, and bananas, often work best. Wash and section fruit in advance so it's ready to eat when you are.

Fresh fruit is refreshing, sweet, relatively low in calories, and generally rich in both nutrients and fiber. It does contain natural sugar, but because of the fiber content, this is in no way harmful. Fruit makes a good A.M. or P.M. snack, and is good in combination with nonfat yogurt and/or cereals, or blended in with crushed ice and orange juice for a deliciously filling smoothie.

Fresh vegetables. Prewashed baby carrots; slices of green pepper, yellow pepper, red pepper, cucumber, fennel, or celery; alfalfa or other bean sprouts; snow peas; raw green beans, wax beans; and soy bean pods (edamame) are great. Vegetables are crunchy and satisfying to chew; they are generally very low in calories, and high in nutrients and fiber. Prewashed and packaged baby carrots are especially convenient. Vegetables make a good P.M. snack, and can be combined with nutritious dips, such as hummus. Vegetables (without dip) make the very best choice for "idle" snacking, or snacking from boredom, because they are very nutritious, but very low in calories.

Whole-grain or multigrain breads. Varieties without added oil or butter are best, to be eaten without spreads; whole-wheat, oat bran, or multigrain bagels.

Breads are not low in calories, but whole-grain breads without spreads are very filling and nutritious. Adding spreads, such as margarine, butter, or cream cheese is not recommended, as this adds lots of fat and calories. Breads with seeds and nuts are higher in calories, but also tend to be more filling and nutritious; they make for a hearty and satisfying snack. All-fruit spreads are reasonable additions. Breads make good A.M. or P.M. snacks, and are good in combination with dried fruit, all-fruit preserves, some fresh fruits, and nutritious dips such as humus.

Cereals. Cereals should be high in fiber, low in added sugar, salt, and fat. Easily held, large-morsel cereals, such as Post Spoon Size Shredded Wheat, Quaker Toasted Oat Squares, Barbara's Puffins, or Shredded Spoonfuls make for convenient snacking. Good choices for eating alone, or mixing in nonfat yogurt; nonfat granolas; oat bran O's or flakes; various varieties of multigrain flakes; Grapenuts; and muesli. See Resource 4 for more product recommendations.

Cereals can be eaten alone, or mixed with yogurt. Cereals with small morsels, such as muesli or granola, are best for mixing; those with large morsels or clusters are best for snacking. Cereals are fiber-rich and filling, crunchy, and satisfying. Packed in a zip-lock bag, a cereal mix is a great thing to snack on throughout the day.

Dried fruit. Raisins, apricots, dates, figs, peaches, pears, and whole bananas (avoid banana chips) are available dried. Choose dried fruit without added sugar. Dried fruit is not "low-calorie," but it is very nutritious and filling. The removal of water from the fruit makes for a snack that is packed with fiber and nutrients. A wide variety of dried fruits is available; dried whole bananas, for example, seem to be little known, and although they tend not to look great, they are delicious! Avoid excessive variety on any given day. Dried fruit makes for good A.M. or P.M. snacking, and is good in combination with whole-grain bread. Dried fruit also offers the benefits of convenience, portability, and a long shelf life; you can leave some in a zip-lock bag in your office for a few days if you don't want to carry a snack with you every day.

Chips. Only baked chips are recommended; most chips are high in added oils and calories, and relatively nutrient poor. The Guiltless Gourmet product line is especially recommended; see Resource 4.

Baked chips are crunchy, tasty, and satisfying, but otherwise do not make a great snack. They are easy to overeat, and do not provide the nutrient value of other snack items listed. Snack on baked chips in the afternoon when you feel the need for something salty.

Dips. Dips come in many varieties, and most are not good choices for snacking. Recommended are hummus, nonfat bean dips, nonfat salsa, guacamole, and nonfat chutneys.

Dips make a good P.M. snack in combination with bread, crackers, or chips. However, many dips are high in calories and nutrient poor. Limit your choice to dips made from beans or vegetables, such as hummus (made from chick peas), salsa (made from tomatoes), and guacamole (made from avocado).

Crackers, rice cakes. Whole-grain crackers high in fiber and without added fat are good choices for snacking. Rice cakes are generally low in fat, come in a variety of flavors, and offer a good alternative to crackers. See Resource 4 for specific products recommended.

Crackers come in many varieties, many with added fat, sugar, and/or salt. But well-chosen crackers are high in fiber, nutritious, crunchy, and satisfying. They make a good P.M. snack alone, or in combination with dips or dried fruit. Rice cakes, which tend to be low in fat and calories, are a good alternative.

Nuts, seeds. Almonds, walnuts, peanuts, pecans, pistachios, soy nuts, sunflower seeds. Nuts and seeds are very nutritious, and make a good substitute for foods at mealtime. They also make a convenient snack food. But they are high in fat and calories, and are easy to overeat. Limit snacking on nuts and seeds to small portions of one variety per day. Make sure nuts are replacing other foods, not simply eaten in addition to everything else. When snacking on nuts or seeds, choose those that are dry-roasted, or otherwise prepared without added oil or salt.

Trail mix. This is essentially a combination of dried fruits, nuts, seeds, and cereals. You can make this yourself, or buy premixed varieties. Avoid mixes that include any added sugar or oil, coconut, or chocolate chips.

Trail mixes made only of dried fruits, whole grains, nuts, and seeds are very high in nutritional value, high in fiber, and filling, and thus justify their rather high calorie content. Makes a convenient snack for any time of day.

Dairy. Nonfat yogurts and cottage cheese make a good snack alone, or in combination with dried fruit, fresh fruit, and/or cereals.

Dairy adds a good source of calcium and other nutrients to your snack "repertoire," and goes well with other recommended items. Convenient to carry in single-serve containers. Good for snacking any time of day.

Snack bars. Granola or cereal bars with at least 2 grams of fiber per 100 calories, and without added oils. See Resource 4.

Granola bars and related products combine cereals, nuts, seeds, and dried fruit into a convenient, single-serve package. These bars can be very nutritious, filling, and satisfying, but care must be exercised, as some brands are high in added fat and are essentially "glorified" candy bars. Resource 4 offers brand recommendations.

Other. Nonfat puddings, custards, Jell-O's; apple sauce; and fruit cocktail, for example, are available in single-serve containers—ideal for snacking. See Resource 4. These are convenient snack items that may be especially valuable for promoting healthful snacking in children. Dessert-like snacks should be restricted to the afternoon. Applesauce is a good alternative to yogurt, and can be mixed with cereal or dried fruit; all-natural varieties without added sugar are recommended.

Snack Preparation Tips

- Make snacking easy by choosing "ready to go" items in single-serve containers, such as raisins in a single-serve box, applesauce, fruit cups, yogurt, granola bars, etc.
- Within each category of snack foods, use those that are easiest to prepare and/or to eat on the go. For example, apples and bananas may be quicker and easier to use in snacks than other fruits. As time permits, wash and dice fruits and store them in plastic bags or containers for quick eating.
- Dried fruit is ready to eat, and travels well.
- Prewashed, prepackaged vegetables, such as baby carrots, make a particularly convenient snack.
- Store cereals, nuts, or seeds in resealable bags for easy snacking.

Snack Transportation Tips

Snacks are most valuable if they are always accessible. Store a variety of snacks for each day in an insulated lunch bag, available in most supermarkets and drug stores. Keep the "snack pack" near you in the car, under your desk at work, or in a drawer. Have the various snack items packaged in a way that makes them easy and convenient to get to repeatedly throughout the day.

The Well-timed Snack

- The very thing our mothers warned us about, "....snacking can spoil your appetite!..." is part of what makes snacking so valuable.
- Eat nutritious snacks as you begin to get hungry to keep hunger under control.
- Have a light but nutritious snack before mealtime, or in advance of a social event that might otherwise lead to overeating.
- Snack an hour or so before the end of your workday to be sure to arrive home with your appetite under control. If possible, with your after-work hunger in check, use this time to get in some physical activity before your dinner.
- Establish a pattern to your snacking that helps you to know you can always eat when you get hungry, relieving anxiety often associated with "dieting" efforts.

A Snack Instead

Use nutritious snacks to:

- Reduce portion sizes in your meals.
- Replace less nutritious foods, such as cakes, cookies, muffins, or candy.
- Reduce the amount you eat at social events.
- Avoid eating foods others bring to your workplace.
- Resist the temptation of fast-food restaurants.
- Keep your appetite in check all day, and avoid end-of-day binges.
- Remove high-fat, high-sugar, nutrient-poor foods from your diet.
- Relieve stress, frustration, or boredom as needed.
- Take control of your own "nutritional environment" wherever you go.

Resource 7: The Way to Include Kids in Healthful Eating

Kids are people, too (sort of). And they need to eat! If you have children, your ability to eat well depends in part on their willingness to do so; preparing different meals for everyone in the house is an inconvenience that can destroy even the strongest commitment to dietary health. The dietary pattern that will promote your health offers comparable benefits to your children. Entries here provide guidance for overcoming any resistance your children may have to improvements in the family diet, and for creating a healthful pattern of family eating that includes everyone.

Sharing Good Eating Habits with Children: General Approaches

In our opinion, the challenge of eating well in the modern nutritional environment is something families should face together. For very small children, their eating depends entirely on you; their eating habits will be good if yours are.

As your children grow, if good nutrition matters to you, talk to them about why it matters. Adding nutrition to the list of "coming of age" topics (see Step 4) parents address with children makes good sense to us. Avoid criticism, but make your values and priorities clear. As always when advising your children what you want them to do, it's very important to set a good example. "Do as I say, not as I do" is not an approach that tends to work.

Make your home a safe, but also satisfying, nutritional environment. Eating well is not martyrdom and should not feel like it for you or your kids. Ask your kids what foods they like to have in the house, and use your skills to find the most nutritious alternatives in each category. They can eat the foods they like and still have good nutrition if you communicate, and compromise.

Let your children snack, but set limits on the types of food acceptable for snacking. If they snack on nutritious foods, you don't need to be overly concerned about how much they eat at mealtime. Help them to be at ease with food, eating when they get hungry, stopping when they get full. The more relaxed you are about their overall pattern of eating, the easier it will be to nudge it in the direction you want it to go.

Been There, Done That...

When it comes to offering advice about how to get kids to eat well, you may be thinking, "Easy for them to say!..."

Well, nothing's foolproof, but our recommendations have been rigorously field-tested! Collectively, we are parents to seven children! We've made this work at home; you can too!

Growing up eating well makes eating well come naturally for the rest of your life. Start your children early on the way to good nutrition, and it will lead them to a lifetime of health benefits.

Food Preparation/Nutrition Tips for Content Kids

Breakfast

- If your child eats cereal in the morning and loves all the sugary, colorful, fat-laden ones that he/she sees on TV, start by changing his/her cereal. There are a lot of kid-oriented healthy equivalents out there that are just as tasty, colorful, and cute. We included a few in our recommended products (see the table in Resource 4), but just look to find what might grab him/her in a health food store (or even the supermarket) or better yet, have your child pick it out him/herself. Make sure to serve it with fat-free milk.

- On, let's say, Sunday, make a big bowl of oatmeal that will last your family two or three days and have it ready in a big resealable container for breakfast. You can either warm it up in the microwave with a little milk in the morning, to moisten it back up, or you can eat it cold with a fat-free fruit yogurt or fresh, diced fruit or berries. On Wednesday night, throw together a concoction of fresh fruit yogurt muesli (or any mix of various cereals of your choice) and place in the refrigerator. The exact amounts do not matter; you cannot go wrong with this formula. In the morning, the blend of yogurt, fruit juices, and grains makes for a luscious "creamy" breakfast. That will keep for two days. Another tasty favorite is couscous with fat-free yogurt and raisins with a little sugar. Make the couscous ahead of time and store it plain in a sealed container in the refrigerator. All you need to do when you are ready for breakfast is heat it up in the microwave (or not) and mix it with the yogurt and raisins. It's also nice with hot milk.

- If you have the chance to make pancakes on a weekend morning, make some extras (filled with fresh fruit) and freeze them in individual packs of two or three. It will come in handy on a busy school morning!
- If the kids are used to a glass of chocolate milk in the morning, make sure and use a product such as Ovaltine, Rich Chocolate Flavor (with fat-free milk) rather than chocolate syrup. It's more nutritious and less sugary and tastes very similar to what they are used to.

Lunch Sandwiches

Start with the simplest, least noticeable changes such as:
- Change bread from varieties low in fiber with added partially hydrogenated oils to whole-grain, low-fat varieties.
- Change peanut butter with added partially hydrogenated oils to all natural peanut butter.
- Change jam with added sugar to all-fruit jam of the same flavor.
- Use sliced turkey or chicken instead of bologna or salami on the sandwich. Then start experimenting with sandwich wraps, including thin wheat breads or corn flour tortillas. Make sandwiches by "wrapping" these bread alternatives around a variety of nutritious ingredients. These can be made the night before without losing their flavor. For the kids, these are fun to eat because they are "cool"; and for you, they are a nutritional winner

because you can more readily "hide" a nutritious veggie in them, such as grated carrot (freshly ground in the mini processor, they stay moist and very bright), and be more adventurous with ingredients.

Snacks

Combine fun, convenience, and good nutrition in snacks so that your kids will want them, and you'll be glad they do!

Fill big glass jars, right on your kitchen counter, with healthy snacks that the kids can have access to whenever they get hungry and that are easy to pack when getting their lunches ready in the morning. These all keep well and just need to be replenished from time to time. Make sure the jars have a big enough opening that you can easily reach in all the way to the bottom. Get your snack baggies ready and go!

Jar #1: Filled with a homemade "trail mix" made up of: healthy cereal—the following combination works well: Quaker Toasted Oatmeal Squares, Kashi Strawberry Crisp Pillows, Chocolate Pillows, Apple Pillows, and New Morning Wafflers; chopped dates (Calavo California Dates are nice because they are rolled in oat flour with no added sugar and are bite size); chopped nuts, if your children like them—and they probably will with this concoction; and even a few semi-sweet chocolate chips—just enough to make hunting for them part of the fun!

Having the kids participate in deciding what should go in their trail mix—and adding it in (with your guidance, of course)—makes it more fun and virtually guarantees that they will eat it.

Jar #2: Filled with dried fruit. The mix should be colorful and enticing, and again, placed in plain view. Dried fruits are sweet and chewy and a wide variety is available in most supermarkets. Dried whole bananas are particularly delicious, although funny looking (they look a bit like beef jerky!) and are often overlooked because they are found next to the fresh tropical fruits in the supermarket. (These are not to be mistaken with banana chips, which are usually loaded with fat.)

Jar #3: Filled with fat-free pretzels such as Snyder's of Hanover sourdough or oat bran varieties, or any low-fat, high-fiber cracker the kids prefer.

Jar #4: Filled with homemade chewy granola squares (see Resource 11 for recipe). Again, these are very nutritious, filling, and have no added fat. They are very easy to make; you throw everything in a food processor to prepare them and the kids love to help spread the sticky dough in the pan! One single batch makes fifty-four squares, which go a long way and keep well. And, to keep the kids entertained, these can be made in a wide variety of fruit flavors with great ease.

Also, fresh fruit should always be available at home. The way you present it in their lunch bags should make it easy to eat, and fun to get to. For example:

- Cut a whole kiwi in half, or cut a thick slice of cantaloupe, and give them a plastic spoon to scoop it up with.
- Cut an orange up in quarters so it's ready to go.
- Use an ice cream scooper or melon ball maker to make fun balls of watermelon or other melon.
- Fresh grapes, blueberries, or strawberries are also very easy to pack. Individually packed canned peaches are also good, but be careful to choose the ones that are sweetened with pear juice concentrate, not with "light" or heavy syrup, as these varieties are unnecessarily high in sugar. The same holds true for applesauce. The unsweetened variety is plenty sweet!

Children love to concoct things themselves and dip and add things together; the food industry is obviously aware of this, and packages many children's snacks accordingly. This is why the crackers packaged with partially hydrogenated cheese or peanut butter or the cookies packaged with chocolate frosting, or the yogurts with sprinkles are so popular. Unfortunately, most of these prepackaged build-your-own snack combinations are not nutritious. To satisfy your child's natural inclination to mix and dip, here are some alternatives where you control the combinations:

- Any dry cereal in a container to which the kids add their snack milk at school
- Fat-free yogurt, honey, and cinnamon with a little jar of low-fat granola
- A cut up apple with a little container of unsalted peanut butter or honey

- A piece of whole-grain bread with a little container of all-fruit jam
- Cooked oatmeal with a little container of cut up fruit
- Yogurt with muesli with a little box of raisins
- Baby carrots with a little container of hummus as a dip

A number of other items make good snacks for kids:

- Baked, soft pretzels (in the freezer section at the supermarket) make a quick, chewy snack. Be careful to check for unnecessary fat. A good choice, if available, is SuperPretzel.
- Low-fat string cheese, fat-free puddings, as well as the low-fat drinkable or squeezable yogurts are a good dairy source and are nice and easy to pack.
- If your child has a "salty tooth" and loves cheese, try packing a piece of ready-to-eat marinated tofu (for example, More than Tofu Italian herb) with fat free crackers. It's a great source of protein.
- Fresh popcorn in the microwave (choose the low-fat variety) is fun to make.
- Think of cereal as crackers. For example, New Morning Fruiteos and Cocoa Oatios taste great dry, and are easy to pack in a little plastic bag.
- Avoid the so-called baked snack crackers, such as Goldfish. These crackers have almost no nutritional value, are high in sodium, low in fiber, and almost half of their calories come from fat.
- As for juices, use 100 percent juice and stay away from other juice drinks. These have added sugar that is not only unnecessary, but can get your kids used to higher and higher sugar intake. Pack only little containers of juice. If the kids are still thirsty, they can drink water from the water fountain.
- Fruit snacks in the form of little gummy characters or roll-ups are cute and appealing to kids, but they offer little nutrition with lots of added sugar. Steer clear of these, or choose the all-fruit varieties available in health food stores.

- Be sure to use skim (fat-free) milk. Milk fat is among the leading sources of saturated fat in the diets of American children. Skim milk has all of the nutrients of whole milk, and even more calcium. This is because the calcium is dissolved in the water portion of milk; the portion of milk taken up by fat contains no calcium. If your kids are at all reluctant to drink skim milk, use a brand that has a richer taste, such as Skim Plus or Simply Smart. Avoid products claiming to be especially for kids while containing fat or additives. Also, be alert to the fact that 2% milk has half the fat of whole milk, and even 1% milk has a fair amount of fat; the percentages used on packages are misleading! They refer to percent of weight, not of calories. And, of course, most of the weight of milk is water.
- Build good nutrition into unexpected places with baked corn and potato chips; soy nuts; snow pea pods; etc. Be creative and have fun, while always keeping good nutrition a priority.

Dinner

- One trick that always works with the kids is to make them guess the secret ingredients in a dinner recipe. This introduces them to new dishes and new tastes in a fun way. It keeps them trying until they guess right, and before you know it, they often love the new food.
- Another way to ensure a balanced meal is to have meals that require them to put ingredients together themselves and "build" their own dish. Examples include fajitas, where they have a choice of refried beans, diced tomatoes, yellow rice, shredded cheese, chicken, peppers, onions, and salsa; falafel, with a choice of cucumbers in yogurt sauce, hummus, avocado, tomatoes, and lettuce; and veggie burgers with sliced tomatoes and lettuce.
- There are ways to make nutritious dishes appealing to children, while keeping them appealing to adults. For example,

use a mild-tasting fresh fish, such as tilapia, to help your children learn to like fish (even our two-year-old asks for seconds and thirds!). Use a sauce or marinade that the children can spoon onto a serving themselves, so they have some control over their meal. Incorporate preserves, or honey, in sauces and glazes, as is done in "sweet and sour" sauces, relishes, or chutneys. A hint of sweetness in a sauce will appeal to the tastes of children.

- Try grilled tuna as a family dinner. It is a "meaty" fish that most kids have at least been introduced to, (although probably masked by mayonnaise) through sandwiches. Grilled swordfish is also a "meaty" favorite. Great with corn on the cob.
- Kids like burgers, but there's no law that they have to be made from beef! Try veggie burgers, turkey burgers, or salmon burgers.
- Do not forget to include salad with most meals; kids get used to this being part of the dinner. If we forget a salad, our kids actually ask for one!

Nutrition "No-No's"

Parents have worried about what and how much their children eat…ever since there have been parents and children! However, much of the time-honored worry relates to making sure that children eat enough. As discussed in Step 4, we often still react as if there is a danger of children eating too little even when the far more likely danger is of them eating too much.

If you don't supervise your children's nutrition at all, it can lead to bad eating habits for them. But too much attention to the wrong things, such as weight, can be even worse. In trying to help your children resist the childhood obesity epidemic, you want to avoid making them feel ashamed or like failures if their weight gets a bit higher than you, or they, might like.

Here is our list of common parenting behaviors you want to avoid as you try to bring your children along with you on the *way to eat*:

- Avoid rewarding eating with dessert. There is no evidence that the "you only get dessert if you finish your dinner" approach results in better eating. Instead, make dinners that are nutritious, provide snacks that are nutritious, and make available desserts that are nutritious as well. When your home is a "safe" nutritional environment, anything your kids eat there will be "good" for them.

- Avoid encouraging plate cleaning. Encourage your children to stop eating when they feel full. You can avoid waste by giving them smaller portions, and refilling their plates if they do clean them and are still hungry. Learning to eat past the point of satiety (fullness) is a very bad habit, and contrary to folklore, doesn't do any good for the starving children of the world!

- Do not expect or require your children to eat the same amount, or types of food, every day. When children have access to healthful, balanced nutrition, they tend to have good eating habits overall, but not necessarily every day. Some days, they may eat very little, other days they won't stop eating. Let this happen naturally. Letting your children get comfortable with eating when hungry, and what they are hungry for, is a good way of defending them against bad eating habits so many of us wind up with.

- Avoid "food fights" with your child. In other words, don't insist that they try new foods, or eat something they don't like. If your child is a "fussy" eater, provide the most nutritious foods you can that they like. A comfortable, relaxed relationship with food will be more important to the health of your child over time than whether or not they ate Brussels sprouts at age four!

- Do not criticize your child's weight. Encourage healthful eating and physical activity, and set a good example. But then help your child not to focus on weight by not focusing on it yourself. If your child tends to be overweight, eating well and being active are the best defenses. Parental criticism does not help, and can be very damaging to self-esteem, which in fact will make weight control even more difficult.

Resource 8: The Way to Eat Out

If you eat out often, the nutritional composition of restaurant, cafeteria, or take-out foods can have a major impact on the quality and content of your overall diet. These entries provide the guidance you need to make sure that when you eat "out," you still remain "in" the bounds of a healthful way of eating.

Restaurant Selection Guide

In general, you will do well to choose restaurants that:

- Offer a variety of dishes made with whole-grain products (e.g., pasta), fish, seafood, vegetables, and/or poultry.
- Offer dishes that are grilled, baked, broiled, or poached rather than fried.
- Are willing to modify dishes to satisfy your preferences, such as reducing the fat content.
- Indicate nutritious or "heart-healthy" choices on the menu.
- Offer a variety of vegetable salads.
- Tend to use low-fat sauces, such as vinaigrettes, wine sauces, citrus-juice sauces, and tomato sauces.
- Provide adequate, but not excessive, portions.

Avoid restaurants that:

- Serve only, or mostly, fried food.
- Will not modify dishes to suit your preferences.
- Use mostly cream, or cheese-based sauces.
- Offer buffets or "all-you-can-eat" options.
- Provide especially large portions.
- Do not indicate nutritious, heart-healthy, or low-calorie/ low-fat options on the menu.

At Italian restaurants, choose pasta, fish, seafood, or poultry dishes with tomato, olive-oil, or wine-based sauces; avoid excessive cheese, cream sauces, or meat.

At Chinese restaurants, choose vegetarian, tofu, seafood, and poultry dishes; ask for low-oil preparation.

At Mexican restaurants, be careful to avoid too much cheese or fried food, including the tortilla chips. Choose soft tortillas instead of hard taco shells. Look, or ask, for nonfat refried beans.

At French restaurants, be careful to avoid excessive cream, butter, or cheese. Try to select restaurants offering Southern French, or Provencal, cooking, which tends to be much lighter than Northern French cuisine.

At delis, choose whole-grain breads and lean cold cuts such as sliced turkey breast. Avoid fatty, highly processed meats, such as pastrami or corned beef. Use mustard instead of butter or mayonnaise.

At grills and diners, generally avoid fried foods and burgers; take advantage of the wide selection to choose salads (avoid cheese and croutons), vegetable side dishes, fish, poultry, pasta, or vegetarian dishes.

Limit visits to, or avoid, fast-food restaurants. If you do frequent these.

Fast-food Restaurant Guide

In many ways, the best advice about fast-food restaurants is to avoid them altogether. Most offer selections that are very high in fat and calories, high in saturated and trans fat, high in sugar or salt, and very limited in nutritional value.

But, fast-food restaurants are convenient and inexpensive, and you may find them irresistible from time to time. Even as you work to reduce the role of fast-food restaurants in your diet, use the following information to improve the choices you make.

- Don't drive through unless there is a good reason, such as a hail storm! The "drive through" combines fast-food eating with no physical activity; at least get out of the car to stretch your legs.
- Choose franchises that offer and identify nutritious dishes, such as Subway, rather than franchises that specialize in burgers or fried foods.
- Avoid deep fried foods whenever possible.
- At any fast-food restaurant or franchise you intend to visit repeatedly, ask to see the calorie and nutritional content of the dishes you order. Best to know!
- Avoid the temptation to go for large or "super" portion sizes. These offer more food for the dollar, but they also provide more calories, more fat, more salt, and more sugar. Is it really a bargain to gain weight inexpensively?

- Choose water instead of soda; sodas add many empty calories to a meal.
- Always make a salad with low-fat dressing a part of your meal if possible.
- Always add extra vegetables to your meal (e.g., sliced lettuce, tomato, onion) when possible; avoid additions such as cheese or bacon.

The nutritional composition of foods at leading fast-food restaurants is available at: www.fatcalories.com.

In summary, if you cannot, or do not choose to, avoid fast-food restaurants, prioritize those that offer salads and freshly prepared foods; use cooking methods other than frying; and that post, or at least can provide you, nutritional information about their food.

Menu/Food Ordering Guide

You probably eat out for a well-deserved break, and for recreation. It may be something you do with friends. If you eat out often, the choices you make can influence your overall nutrition, so they are important. But the selection of healthful dishes needs to be balanced with the fun! You will want to get at some important information about menu items, without feeling as though you are interrogating your waiter or waitress.

The best start, as noted above, is to choose a restaurant that provides reasonably healthful dishes to begin with. If you eat regularly at a restaurant where all of the dishes are unhealthy, making healthful selections will be unpleasant at best, impossible at worst. Eat at such restaurants rarely if at all, and go more often to those that make identifying dishes that are nutritious as well as delicious less of a challenge.

Once in the "right" kind of restaurant, here are the important steps to combine a good time, a good meal, and good nutrition.

Questions to Ask

About the menu in general:

    1) Do you have any dishes that are especially healthy that you recommend?

    2) Does the menu give complete information about what's in a dish?

3) Is the chef/cook willing to modify dishes to make them healthier?

About a specific dish:

1) What's in the sauce of this dish? Does it contain butter, cream, or cheese?

2) Is this dish rich, or light in your opinion?

3) Is there any important ingredient in this dish that's not listed, such as cream, cheese, or meats?

Items to Look for on the Menu

Choose:

- dishes that are grilled, baked, broiled, or poached.
- dishes identified as nutritious or heart-healthy.
- lean meats, fish, or vegetarian dishes.
- dishes with light sauces, often made with juices, broth, or vinegar and herbs.
- a salad to accompany your entrée.

Avoid:

- foods that are fried.
- meats that tend to be fatty.
- cream or butter sauces.
- dishes with added cheese.

Requests You Should Consider Making

- Replace butter with olive oil.
- Replace cream sauces with marinara, vinaigrette, olive oil, or wine-based sauces.
- Grill, bake, or broil fish or poultry instead of frying.
- Place the sauce on the side.

Habits You Should Acquire

- Drink water before and during your meal.
- Eat at a leisurely pace.
- Always have salad.
- Avoid the use of butter on bread; eat fresh bread plain.
- Avoid buffets, other than all-vegetable salad bars.

Resource 9: *The Way to Achieve and Maintain a Healthy Weight*

You do not directly control your weight. Weight represents the balance between the food energy, or calories, you take in, and the three processes that burn calories: resting energy expenditure (basal metabolism), physical activity, and heat loss known as postprandial thermogenesis. An understanding of energy balance, and a realistic approach to weight regulation, is essential to long-term weight control.

Please recall the basic weight control philosophy of *The Way to Eat*: eat well, and be physically active. Focus on health, rather than weight, and let a healthful lifestyle take care of your weight. Keep track of your weight not as a primary focus, but just as a "reality check" to make sure you are not overlooking calories or overestimating your physical activity. If you are eating better and being more active, you are succeeding, whatever your weight.

The Body Mass Index (BMI)

The body mass index is one of the standard ways of assessing weight relative to height, and is used by professionals as a guide in weight control efforts. The National Institutes of Health define a body mass index of less than 25 as normal weight; 25–29.9 as overweight; 30–34.9 as stage I obesity; 35–39.9 as stage II obesity; and 40 or higher as stage III obesity.

Your body mass index is your weight in kilograms, divided by your height measured in meters, and squared. As a formula, the BMI is:

$$kg/m2$$

A kilogram, or kg, is 2.2 pounds; a pound is 0.45 kilograms. A meter is 39.37 inches, or 3.28 feet. To determine your weight in kilograms, divide your weight in pounds by 2.2. To determine your height in meters, divide your height in inches by 39.37. An example is shown below:

Weight in pounds = 140
Height = 5 ft, 7 in = 67 in

Weight in kilograms = 140/2.2 = 63.6 kg
Height in meters = 67/39.37 = 1.70

BMI = 63.6/(1.70²) = 63.6/2.89 = 22

Be aware that the BMI cannot "tell" the difference between fat and muscle; it simply provides a measure of weight relative to height. If you have a very large or very small frame, or a particularly large or small muscle mass, the BMI may not accurately reflect your level of thinness of fatness. This is a limitation to its use.

Determining Your Body-Mass Index (BMI)

Height in feet and inches is shown across the top, weight in pounds is shown in the left-hand column. Each entry in the table represents the BMI for a particular combination of height and weight. BMIs that represent the transition points from lean to overweight (25), from overweight to obese (30), and from one stage of obesity to the next (35, 40) are shown in bold. BMI values are close approximations due to rounding. BMI values in the recommended or "healthiest" range are shaded in gray. Note that if you are very slight, or very muscular, your BMI might fall above or below the shaded area and still be consistent with excellent health.

Height in Feet & Inches

	4'10"	5'	5'2"	5'4"	5'6"	5'8"	5'10"	6'	6'2"	6'4"
100	21	20	18	<18	<18	<18	<18	<18	<18	<18
110	23	21.5	20	19	<18	<18	<18	<18	<18	<18
120	25	23.5	22	21	19	18	<18	<18	<18	<18
130	27	25	24	22	21	20	19	<18	<18	<18
140	29	27	26	24	23	21	20	19	18	<18
150	31	29	27.5	26	24	23	22	20	19	18
160	33.5	31	29	27.5	26	24	23	22	20.5	19.5
170	36	33	31	29	27.5	26	24	23	22	21
180	38	35	33	31	29	27	26	24.5	23	22
190	40	37	35	33	31	29	27	26	24.5	23
200	>40	39	37	34	32	30	29	27	26	24
210	>40	41	38	36	34	32	30	28.5	27	26
220	>40	>40	40	38	36	33	32	30	28	27
230	>40	>40	>40	40	37	35	33	31	30	28
240	>40	>40	>40	>40	39	37	34.5	33	31	29
250	>40	>40	>40	>40	40	38	36	34	32	30.5
260	>40	>40	>40	>40	>40	40	37	35	33	32
270	>40	>40	>40	>40	>40	>40	39	37	35	33
280	>40	>40	>40	>40	>40	>40	40	38	36	34
290	>40	>40	>40	>40	>40	>40	>40	39	37	35
300	>40	>40	>40	>40	>40	>40	>40	41	39	37

Weight in Pounds

Weight Loss/Maintenance Guidelines

- In general, the best approach to weight loss is to focus on eating well and being physically active rather than on weight per se. Think about health more, and about weight less. Remember that you can "choose" what to eat, and how active to be; you cannot simply choose what to weigh.

- Eating well means choosing foods that make up a healthful dietary pattern, rich in grains, fruits, and vegetables, and making sure portions are reasonable, and total calories are appropriate.

- Physical activity is vital to long-term weight control. Accumulating at least thirty minutes of moderate physical activity on most days, every week, is encouraged.

- If committed to weight loss, select a moderate and sustainable pace. We recommend that you not lose more than 2 pounds per week, as rapid weight loss tends to be rapidly reversible, and may also pose some health threats.

- To lose 1 pound per week, take in 500–600 fewer calories per day than you need for weight maintenance. To lose 2 pounds per week, take in 1,000 fewer calories per day. We encourage slow, steady weight loss at a rate of 1/2–1 pound per week; this requires reducing daily calories by a much more manageable 250–300 per day. Recognize that losing just 1/2 pound per week would result in a 26 pound weight loss if maintained for a year!

- Expect to hit "plateaus" as you lose weight. This is because basal metabolic rate, and calorie needs, go down as weight goes down. Resist this tendency by being physically active. Physical activity tends to increase basal metabolism.

- The more you need to restrict calories to lose weight, the more important it is to eat a healthful variety of foods. Also, the potential value of a multivitamin/mineral supplement increases the more you restrict your total daily calorie intake.

- The *way to eat* is also the way to lose and control weight. Avoid "dieting." Instead, improve your way of eating, and your weight will tend to take care of itself.
- Check your weight every one to two weeks to gauge your progress, and to make sure your assessments of activity level and calorie intake are accurate. But do not let the scale be your measure of success. If you are eating better, and/or being more physically active, you have succeeded even if the scale is not telling you exactly what you would like to hear.

Determining Your Daily Calorie Needs for Weight Maintenance or Loss

Everyone's calorie needs are unique. The only way to know exactly how many calories you need per day to maintain or lose weight is for you to undergo some very elaborate testing on a metabolic ward in a nutrition research center. Even then, the "answer" would only be correct as long as your weight and activity level stayed constant.

Fortunately, some fairly accurate approximations can be reached with very simple approaches—no technology required! Presented here are two methods of estimating your calorie, or food energy, needs under varying circumstances. The first is simpler, but slightly less accurate. The second involves just a bit more math, but gets you closer to the truth. Use whichever suits you to get a reasonable sense of your food energy needs— a helpful starting point for portion control, and weight regulation.

Method 1

This is a relatively simple method for determining your energy needs for maintaining your current weight based upon your weight in kilograms, and your activity level.

To find out your weight in kilograms, divide your current weight in pounds by 2.2 (one pound = 2.2 kilograms).

Determine your activity level:

Sedentary: office work, no regular exercise

Moderate: activity, such as walking, a few times a week

Active: consistent exercise for at least 30 minutes, 5 to 7 times a week

Then identify your energy needs using the following chart:

Energy Needs for Weight Maintenance

	Sedentary	Moderate	Active
Overweight BMI over 25	20–25 kcal/kg	30 kcal/kg	35 kcal/kg
"Normal" weight BMI of 18-25	30 kcal/kg	35 kcal/kg	40 kcal/kg
Underweight BMI under 18	30 kcal/kg	40 kcal/kg	45–50 kcal/kg

For weight loss, first figure out the calories you need to maintain your current weight, then subtract 500 calories/day. This calorie level will allow you to lose weight at a safe rate of approximately 1 pound a week, although you will eventually "plateau" when weight loss causes your basal metabolic rate to fall. You can compensate for this by basing your calorie needs for a 1lb/week rate of weight loss on your new weight.

Here's an example:

Mary is 5'2" and weighs 150 pounds. Using the BMI table, Mary's BMI is 27. Her weight in kilograms is 150 pounds divided by 2.2, or 68 kg. She walks for thirty minutes about two to three times a week, which would be considered moderate activity. Using the chart above, Mary's energy needs would be 30 calories per kilogram, or 2,040 calories a day to maintain her weight. Since Mary would like to get her BMI to 25 or below for a healthier weight, she needs to subtract 500 calories a day. Mary now needs 1,540 calories a day to achieve a weight loss of about 1 pound a week. At this calorie level, Mary can lose approximately 15 pounds in about four months, although she may need to adjust slightly along the way to account for the plateau effect.

Method 2

(For those devoted to accuracy and unintimidated by mathematics!)

The Harris-Benedict Equation uses age, height, and weight to estimate basal energy expenditure (BEE), the minimum amount of energy needed by your body for weight maintenance.

For Women:

BEE (kcal/day) = 66.5 + (13.8 x W) + (5.0 x H) – (6.8 x A)

For Men:

BEE (kcal/day) = 655.1 + (9.6 x W) + (1.8 x H) – (4.7 x A)

Where:

W = weight in kilograms (weight in pounds divided by
2.2 = weight in kilograms)

H = height in centimeters (height in inches multiplied by
2.54 = height in centimeters)

A = age in years

The BEE value is then multiplied by an activity factor to estimate the daily calories you need to maintain your current weight.

Activity Factor	Description of Activities
Very Light = 1.3 for women and men	seated and standing activities, driving, cooking, playing a musical instrument
Light = 1.5 for women, 1.6 for men	golf, sailing, housecleaning, child care, walking 2.5–3 mph
Moderate = 1.6 for women, 1.7 for men	dancing, skiing, tennis, cycling, walking 3.5–4 mph
Heavy = 1.9 for women, 2.1 for men	basketball, football, soccer, climbing

Here's an example:

Jack is thirty-five years old, 6'2" and weighs 220 pounds. He is a carpenter by trade, skis when he can, and rides a bike three times a week.

First, the conversions:

Weight: 220 pounds divided by 2.2 = 100 kilograms (kg)

Height: 6'2" = 74 inches multiplied by 2.54 = 188 centimeters (cm)

Now, plug them into the BEE formula for men:

BEE = 655.1 + (9.6 x 100 kg) + (1.8 x 188 cm) - (4.7 x 35)

BEE = 1790 calories a day needed for Jack's body at rest

Next, adjust the BEE for activity level, which for Jack would be moderate.

1790 BEE calories times 1.7 = 3,000 calories a day for weight maintenance.

Even though Jack's BMI is 28, he has a muscular build and is happy with his appearance. Jack can enjoy 3,000 calories a day as long as he maintains his activity level.

In summary, to estimate daily calories to:

Maintain weight: BEE formula times activity factor.

Lose weight: BEE formula times activity factor minus 500 calories a day.

Gain weight: BEE formula times activity factor plus 500 calories a day.

Portion Size Guide

Weight control depends not only on what you eat, but also on how much. Excess calories can come from almost any food source if portions are too big. Use this table as a basis to gauge serving sizes in various food categories, and to help establish a realistic frame of reference for the size of the meals and dishes you eat. Keep in mind, if your drinks, meals, snacks, or sandwiches are routinely super-sized, they are apt to share that characteristic with you!

Food Group	Standard Serving Size
Whole grains	1 slice bread; ½–1 cup breakfast cereal; ½ cup cooked cereal, grains, or pasta
Fruits	1 medium piece of fresh fruit; 4 ounces of 100% fruit juice; ½ cup canned, cooked, or chopped fruit; ½ cup dried fruit; about one small handful
Vegetables	½ cup cooked vegetables; 1 cup raw vegetable or salad; 6 ounces vegetable juice; ½ cup is about the size of a tennis ball; 1 cup is about the size of your fist
Vegetable oils and added fats	1 teaspoon oil; ⅛ avocado; 1 tablespoon salad dressing; 1 teaspoon soft margarine
Nuts and seeds	1 ounce or ½ cup; 1 tablespoon peanut or almond butter, about the size of the tip of your thumb
Beans and legumes	½ cup cooked beans, lentils, or peas; ½ cup tofu; 1 cup soymilk
Fish, chicken, turkey beef, pork, lamb	3 ounces cooked, about the size of a deck of cards
Dairy	1 cup milk or yogurt; 1 ½ ounces low-fat cheese, about the size of four stacked dice; ½ cup ricotta cheese

Frequently Overlooked Calories

As discussed in Steps 1 and 4, there are certain foods and sources of calories to which many of us tend to be inattentive. Overlooking calories is a particularly important issue if you are trying to lose weight.

Be especially attentive to the following foods and beverages during weight-loss efforts. Overlooking any of these common items could be the reason why you think you should be losing weight, but are not.

Beverages
- Alcoholic beverages: wine, beer, liquor
- Soft drinks, sodas

Condiments
- Cream/milk in coffee
- Croutons
- Grated cheese
- Sugar in coffee

Dressings
- Bleu cheese dressing
- Creamy salad dressing

Snacks
- Candies
- Chips
- Crackers
- Nuts

Spreads
- Butter
- Cream cheese
- Margarine
- Mayonnaise

Sauces
- Butter- or cheese-based sauces
- Cream-based sauces

Other
- Kids' leftover food scraps
- Eating while cooking or baking

Critique of Commercial Weight-loss Programs

- Overall, there is limited evidence that any commercial weight-loss programs produce sustainable weight loss.
- The best predictor of long-term maintenance of weight loss is the combination of a dietary pattern high in complex carbohydrates and regular physical activity. Participation in a commercial weight-loss program is not known to increase the likelihood of long-term success with weight control.
- The commercial weight-loss industry in the United States was investigated by Congress in the 1990s. As a result, any credible program should offer you a written summary of typical results achieved. Don't enroll in a program that will not make such information available upon request.
- Commercial weight loss in the U.S. is a multibillion-dollar industry. With all of the people and all of the money involved, it is that much more noteworthy that clear evidence of long-term benefit is for the most part lacking.
- Leading weight-loss programs either provide meals, or provide instruction in choosing foods. Before using a program that provides you with meals, address two important issues. 1) Is the cost of the program justified by what you are getting out of it? and, 2) What will you do when the program stops providing you with meals? In general, don't use programs unless they provide instruction in skills that you can make use of long-term.
- Avoid any commercial weight-loss program that is built around a "fad" or unbalanced diet.
- Programs that promote weight control through healthful eating are preferred. The Weight Watchers points program is an example. We support use of this program as needed.
- If considering a commercial weight-loss program, consult your health-care provider, and ideally, a dietitian for advice.

Medications & Supplements

Medications

- There are two basic categories of medication for weight loss: over-the-counter (OTC) drugs and prescription drugs.
- There are many over-the-counter drugs for weight loss, too many to mention by name. Most are stimulant drugs, related to the amphetamines; others affect brain chemicals called neurotransmitters. These drugs either suppress appetite, increase metabolism, or both.
- As of 2002, there are only two prescription weight-loss drugs approved by the United States Food and Drug Administration: sibutramine, marketed as Meridia, and orlistat, marketed as Xenical. Sibutramine raises levels of two neurotransmitters in the brain: serotonin, and nor-epinephrine. Orlistat interferes with fat absorption in the intestines.
- There is some risk involved in the use of any drug for weight loss. In general, medication use is only appropriate if the benefits of medication use clearly outweigh the risks. This is more likely to be the case when you are very obese rather than slightly overweight, and when other approaches to weight control are not working. Under any circumstances, use of medication for weight loss should be discussed with your health-care provider, and as needed, a dietitian. Don't decide to use medication on your own.
- Some weight-loss medications have been shown to help with weight loss in the short-term, but none has been studied over years and decades. More and more obesity experts believe that weight control may need to be treated with medication the way high blood pressure, diabetes, or high cholesterol are treated, chronically, or even permanently. Medication for diabetes is not stopped when the blood sugar becomes normal—this is merely evidence that the medication is working! Yet, in weight control, most people tend to stop medication

once weight is lost. This generally results in the weight being regained.

- Weight-loss medication, when needed at all, is probably needed long-term. But the safety of weight-loss medication for long-term use is not known. Given these two important issues, the role of medication in the control of weight should be limited.

The way to use weight control medications in general is as follows:

- Only with the advice of a physician or other health-care professional
- Only to enhance, never to replace, the role of eating well and being physically active
- In combination with dietary counseling from a dietitian

Supplements

- Dietary supplements for weight loss, including herbs, nutrients, and combination products, are far more numerous, and far less regulated, than drugs. As a result, such products range from potentially useful, to harmless but useless, to truly dangerous.
- There are many wild claims about the dramatic benefits from weight-loss supplements. Most of these sound too good to be true—and are, in fact, not true. There is no supplement that safely and reliably leads to lasting weight loss.
- Many supplements are promoted with "testimonials," great success stories told by thrilled customers. In our view, here is how you should think of these stories if, indeed, they are true at all. Every now and then we all hear a news story that is amazing, such as a baby falling out of a building, and suffering only a scratch. From this, we do not conclude that it is safe for babies to fall out of buildings! We think: wow, that's unusual and amazing. Testimonials are also the "unusual," "amazing," or short-term results, not the usual result. They do not provide useful information.
- Supplements chosen carefully with the guidance of a health-care or nutrition professional, such as a doctor or

dietitian, may offer benefits on occasion. For example, chromium supplementation may be beneficial in insulin resistance. Consult with a trusted professional before deciding to use supplements in support of weight-loss goals.

- When restricting calories to try and lose weight, supplementing vitamins and minerals for general health promotion may be appropriate.
- Remember that the people advertising supplements to you are selling something!

Energy Expenditure for Physical Activity

The following table shows energy expenditure associated with various activities in terms of METs, which are multiples of the basal, or resting metabolic rate, and in calories (kcal) per minute. The basal metabolic rate (BMR) varies with body size, so the numbers shown are estimates. Resting metabolic rate represents the energy expended by basal metabolism while not involved in any physical activity. The calories "burned" by an activity can be determined by multiplying the calories burned per minute of the activity, multiplied by the number of minutes spent doing the activity, and then subtracting the calories that were used for basal metabolism during that same time.

For example, walking slowly burns roughly 3 kcal/minute. So, walking slowly for 30 minutes burns 3 x 30, or 90 kcal. During that same 30 minutes, basal metabolism burns roughly 1.5 kcal minute, or 1.5 x 30, or 45 kcal. The calories "burned" by walking are 90–45, or 45 kcal.

Activity	Multiples of the Basal Metabolic Rate ("METs")	Calories Burned per Minute
Resting (sitting or lying down)	1.0	1.2–1.7
Sweeping	1.5	1.8–2.6
Driving (car)	2.0	2.4–3.4
Walking slowly (2 mph)	2.0–3.5	2.8–4

Activity	Multiples of the Basal Metabolic Rate ("METs")	Calories Burned per Minute
Bicycling slowly (6 mph)	2.0–3.5	2.8–4
Horseback riding (walk)	2.5	3–4.2
Volleyball	3.0	3.5
Mopping	3.5	4.2–6.0
Golf	4.0–5.0	4.2–5.8
Swimming slowly	4.0–5.0	4.2–5.8
Walking moderately fast (3 mph)	4.0–5.0	4.2–5.8
Baseball	4.5	5.4–7.6
Bicycling moderately fast (12 mph)	4.5–9.0	6–8.3
Dancing	4.5–9.0	6–8.3
Skiing	4.5–9.0	6–8.3
Skating	4.5–9.0	6–8.3
Walking fast (4.5 mph)	4.5–9.0	6–8.3
Swimming moderately fast	4.5–9.0	6–8.3
Tennis (singles)	6.0	7.7
Chopping wood	6.5	7.8–11
Shoveling	7.0	8.4–12
Digging	7.5	9–12.8
Cross country skiing	7.5–12	8.5–12.5
Jogging	7.5–12	8.5–12.5
Football	9.0	9.1
Basketball	9.0	9.8
Running	15	12.7–16.7
Running, 4 minute mile pace	30	36–51
Swimming (crawl) fast	30	36–51

Adapted from: Katz, D.L., *Nutrition in Clinical Practice*. Philadelphia, PA: Lippincott Williams & Wilkins, 2000. Reprinted with Permission of the Publisher.

Resource 10: The Way to Bake and Cook

For the skills and strategies, knowledge and power, of the *way to eat* to serve you well, they have to work "where the rubber hits the road," or where your fork hits your food! In other words, you need to know how to prepare the foods you will be eating. Provided here are the methods and techniques you need for preparing food that is just as delicious, but much more nutritious, than ever before.

Recommended Cooking Methods

In addition to the ingredients used for preparing food, the methods used can influence the nutritional composition.

Recommended Cooking Methods

- Grilling: does not add fat to food, and can even allow fat in food to drain out. Charring or blackening food, however, can produce carcinogens, and should be avoided.
- Baking: does not add fat to food, and avoids charring.
- Broiling: does not add fat to food, and allows for even cooking.
- Poaching: locks in subtle flavors, and tenderizes dishes. It adds no fat.
- Steaming: fat-free method that is especially good for lightly cooking vegetables.
- Sautéing, or stir-frying: good substitute for frying. Uses less oil, adds less fat, but still allows for the browning or crisping of foods.
- Pressure-cooking: allows for slow, convenient cooking of soups and stews.

Recommended Cooking Equipment

A few key pieces of kitchen equipment can make healthful food preparation easier, more nutritious, and more convenient.

- Small food processor for daily use (optional)
- Large food processor
- Juicer
- Steamer

- Garlic press
- Scissors for cooking use only
- Nonstick pans and pots (reduce oil use), a nonstick baking pan with a removable rim
- Oil mister (allows for reduced oil use)
- Bread maker: mixes are available that allow for convenient preparation of nutritious, home-baked breads
- Crock-Pot
- Pressure cooker
- Grill/grilling machine (e.g., George Foreman models)
- Large see-through, wide-mouthed glass jars

Recommended Ingredient Substitutions

Ingredient substitutions for cooking and baking can be used for virtually any recipe or dish. This approach to improving nutrition is of great value because it allows you to preserve the familiar taste and appearance of dishes you like, while improving the nutrition.

The best substitutes for any given dish are a matter of personal preference, and reaching a decision may involve some trial and error. Keep in mind that while most dishes stand up very well, or are even improved by ingredient substitutions, the occasional dish only tastes good if the original recipe is followed. In that case, recall that it is the nutritional composition of your overall diet, not of any one dish, that is important to your health. Use ingredient substitutions to transform and improve your overall nutrition, while setting the limits that keep your "accept no substitute!" recipes just as they've always been.

To Remove/Reduce	When You Are	The Following	
Fat (Total Saturated, and/or Trans)	**Cooking**	Sauces	
		Glazes	
		Soups/Stews	
		Poultry	
	Baking	Breads	
		Cookies	
		Cakes	

Replace	With
Butter	Olive oil
Cream	"Roux" made up of olive oil/flour paste; whisked with hot milk/broth and/or wine Skim buttermilk
Whole milk	Skim milk
Regular broth, meat stock, butter	Currants simmered in chicken broth Honey/mustard/lemon/curry All-fruit jam, or orange or apple juice concentrate mixed with beer & mustard
Regular broth	Fat-free broth
Skin	Combo of fat-free yogurt/mustard/ concentrated orange juice with garlic powder/paprika/bread crumbs with light olive oil spray
Butter	Olive oil or nothing at all!
Butter/Margarine with Trans Fatty Acids (hydrogenated margarine)	Combo of nonhydrogenated margarine & mashed banana or Apple sauce or Defatted peanut butter
Butter	Canola oil
Sour Cream	Fat-free yogurt
Whole Eggs	Egg whites

To Remove/Reduce	When You Are	The Following	
Fat (Total Saturated, and/or Trans)	**Baking**	Cakes	
		Frostings	
		Pie Crust	
		Crisps/Cobblers	
	Using	Spreads for Sandwiches	

Replace	With
Whole milk	Skim milk
Cream cheese	Combo of part-skim Ricotta cheese and Reduced-fat cream cheese
Butter or heavy cream	Small amount of hot skim milk with bittersweet chocolate melted in Heated all-fruit jams alone or with melted chocolate Fresh fruit and dusting of Confectioner's Sugar
Milk chocolate	Bittersweet chocolate
Butter/Shortening	Canola oil or combo of ground nuts and egg whites
Butter	Combo of ground nuts, apple butter & egg whites
Mayonnaise, Margarine, or Butter	Fat-free yogurt/mustard/lemon juice and curry Basil pesto with or without yogurt Mashed cooked garlic Mustard Hummus Avocado Roasted red peppers (in vinegar) Sundried tomatoes packed in olive oil (washed & drained) Marinated tofu

To Remove/Reduce	When You Are	The Following	
Salt	Cooking	Anything	
	Baking	Anything	
Oil	Frying	Vegetables, fish, chicken, shrimp, etc.	
Sugar	Cooking or Baking	Anything	

Recommended Flavor Enhancers/Seasonings

Instead of cooking with butter, margarine, or frying with oil, experiment with the following to replace fat with flavor!

- Low-fat and low-sodium chicken, beef, or vegetable broth
- Orange or apple juice concentrates
- Unsweetened pineapple juice
- Cooking wines (vermouth, sherry, red)
- All-fruit jam

Replace	With
Salt	Herbs such as thyme, cilantro, onion powder, garlic powder, basil Vinegar Citrus juices (lemon, lime) *Simply reduce the amount of salt used while cooking, and salt individual servings to obtain more salt flavor with less salt use
Salt	Nothing—simply eliminate or reduce the salt & baking soda called for in the recipe
Frying	Coat with fat-free yogurt and sprinkle bread crumbs, and light olive oil spray, and bake at 400°
Sugar	All-fruit preserves/jams Fruit juices Honey *Note that sugar substitutes that are moist and sticky can be used to replace fat as well as sugar in baked goods.*

- Chiles
- Citrus juices, lemon
- Dried fruits
- Freshly minced garlic cloves
- Freshly ground ginger root
- Herbs, fresh and dried: basil, cilantro, rosemary, thyme, chives
- Honey

- Horseradish
- Dried mushrooms
- Mustards
- Capers
- Nuts*
- Pignoli
- Onions, shallots, scallions
- Olives*
- Peppercorns, red pepper flakes
- Salsas
- Spices
- Vinegars: balsamic, cider, red wine, white wine
- Wasabi
- Marinades: wines, low-sodium soy sauce, fruit or vegetable juices

Contain heart-healthy monounsaturated fats but still have many calories; use in small amounts.

Entertainment Tips: Food Preparation for Special Events

- There is no reason why eating well and special occasions cannot go together. As a general strategy, serve dishes that are traditional family favorites, but modify some of the ingredients to improve the nutrition content. This keeps the dishes familiar in taste and appearance, while cutting back on fat and calories. Whenever possible, test such recipe modifications before using them at a special event, because they won't always work!
- If you have family or traditional favorites that cannot be modified, serve them "as is" along with alternatives that are more nutritious. Eating well is about the overall diet, not a single food or dish. If there is a dish you love that simply should not be changed, don't change it: enjoy it!
- Try always to serve plenty of vegetable dishes and salads. Keep sauces and dressings light. Variety and abundance are very festive, and by using grains, pastas, beans, and

vegetables in salads, you can create a spread that is beautiful to look at, delicious to eat, and nutritious!

- Accompany meals with fresh-baked whole-grain breads from local bakeries.
- Replace dips made from sour cream or cheese with more nutritious dips such as hummus, guacamole, bean dips, and salsa. Replace fried chips with baked chips, crisped breads, whole grain crackers, or better still, sliced fresh vegetables.
- Modify dessert recipes to provide choices that are festive and delicious, but reduced in fat and calories.
- Recognize that nutritious eating, cooking, and shopping becomes second nature after a while. Once this happens, preparing festive dishes with good nutrition is easy. Be patient and let it happen. In the mean time, don't allow good nutrition and good times to compete with one another; both are important.

Tips for Efficient Food Preparation

If we had to guess, we would guess that you are busy! Finding time to prepare healthful foods may be as much of a challenge as knowing how. Here are some tips to help you get the most out of what little time you have to prepare nutritious foods for yourself and your family.

- Use knowledge of how to keep a well-stocked pantry (see Resource 5), and how to prepare quick and convenient dishes that provide good nutrition to help you get healthful meals on the table quickly and with little effort.
- Whenever you do have time for food preparation, such as on a weekend, make extra for freezing. It will be a real treat to have a favorite home-cooked meal days or even weeks later, just by defrosting and warming up a dish that's ready to go.
- Use slow-cooking techniques, such as crock pots, that allow you to toss ingredients in a pot in the morning and come home to a slowly simmering soup or stew in the evening.

- Become familiar with preferred brands and products (see Resource 4) so you can make good use of mixes, frozen entrees, and other convenience foods while maintaining good nutrition.

Resource 11: The Way to Plan Meals

Meal Planner Users' Guide

- The meal planner displays a representative distribution of meals and snacks consistent with healthful eating, but not the only one. Many variations on this theme of nutritious eating are possible. Bear in mind that any movement from a less healthful to a more healthful dietary pattern is beneficial to you.

- The foods shown for each day may or may not exactly match the recommended levels of total fat, saturated fat, cholesterol, carbohydrate, and protein. Over time, though, this basic dietary pattern will closely reflect the recommended nutrient levels of the *way to eat*.

- Calorie requirements for weight maintenance vary considerably. Increase or decrease portion sizes, or the frequency of snacks, as appropriate to meet your calorie needs.

- The basic pattern of the planner is based on some assumptions about the average American lifestyle and eating pattern, which may not match your lifestyle. Modify the planner as needed to better fit in with your schedule. The assumptions are as follows:

    1. Time for meal preparation is generally limited.

    2. Dinner is the largest and most social meal of the day. It is also the one meal for which there is some preparation time.

    3. Weekdays are more rushed than weekends. Weekends allow more time, in particular, for breakfast preparation.

    4. Breakfast is often eaten quickly while getting ready for work or school.

    5. Lunch is generally eaten outside the home. Lunch can either be brought from home, or purchased. "Leftovers" from dinner are sometimes used for lunch preparation.

- The amount of variety shown in the planner is moderate, and may be either increased or decreased to match your preferences. As long as your dietary pattern is providing balanced nutrition, you may choose to eat similar foods for particular meals or snacks each day, or to vary from day to day. Maintaining adequate variety in the diet over time is important to health, while avoiding excessive variety in any one meal is important as a means of controlling total calorie intake.

- The planner is not specifically designed for a vegetarian or vegan dietary pattern, but may be adapted to those patterns by substituting plant-based foods for fish and poultry items. Alternatives to "meat" are provided on page 217.

- The planner is intended to provide a basic sense of how to construct a healthful pattern of eating—you do not need to limit yourself to only these foods or this sequence of foods. However, using the foods and sequence of the planner is a good way to get started along the *way to eat*. Once you get comfortable, you can start introducing more variation. Think of this as the "guided tour" of your new, healthy way of eating. Like any guided tour, on this one you need to go where the guide takes you only at first. As soon as you "know your way around," you won't be limited to the "tour route" any more, and can use the basic principles of good eating to chart your own particular *way to eat* well.

Meal or Snack	Recommended Composition
Breakfast	Whole-grain, high-fiber cold cereal, or hot oatmeal with skim milk; nonfat yogurt and/or whole-wheat, or other whole-grain toast, English muffin, or bagel with all-fruit jam and/or fresh fruit any variety, and coffee or tea; nonfat powdered milk in lieu of other creamers, and fruit juice
Weekend Variants	Eggs prepared to taste (without added butter or cheese), whole-grain pancakes, French toast, or waffles (from scratch or nutritious mix)

A.M. Snack   Fresh fruit, any variety; nonfat yogurt; dried fruit; whole-grain bread or cereal

Lunch   Bean, lentil, grain, pasta, or vegetable (mixed green) salad with low-fat vinaigrette or comparable dressing; and/or a sandwich on whole-grain bread or wrap: choose from tuna, turkey, avocado, tomato, lettuce, or any fresh vegetables, hummus, tofu; use nonfat spreads such as mustard, or nutritious spreads such as nut butters (e.g., tahini); limit use of butter, margarine, and mayonnaise; and/or suitable dinner leftovers (soup, stew, chili, any entrée, salad, etc.); and fresh fruit and water, tea, or juice

P.M. Snack   Any A.M. snack item or dry-roasted nuts or seeds; trail mix (mix of dried fruit, nuts, seeds, and whole-grain cereals); baked corn or potato chips; fat-free pretzels; or fresh vegetables (e.g., baby carrots, sliced peppers, tomato wedges, etc.)

Dinner   Mixed green salad with other vegetables (carrots, radishes, tomatoes, sprouts, peppers, onion, cucumber, etc.) to taste; olive oil and vinegar, or vinaigrette dressing without hydrogenated oils; cooked vegetable (corn, broccoli, squash, etc.); and whole-grain bread, or cooked grains; and entrées based often on beans, lentils, fresh fish, or skinless poultry; less often on other meats; use preferred cooking methods and ingredient substitutions for a wide variety of delicious, nutritious sauces; include soups, stews, chilies, and pasta dishes among the options; wine, or beer in moderation as desired

Dessert   Nonfat frozen yogurt or sorbet; and/or fresh fruit (berries, melon, etc.); or; low-fat, store-bought or home-made cookies, cakes, puddings, etc.; use dark chocolate preferentially to milk chocolate

Evening Snack   Avoid, or limit to one item each day. Select from A.M. or P.M. snack choices, or an additional small serving of dessert. Make every effort to conclude all snacking at least two hours prior to your bedtime.

Sample Recipes

The Way to Eat is very expressly not a cookbook. Rather, it provides the skills, strategies, and guidance you need to make the foods and dishes you are used to, or the recipes in any cookbook you like to use, as nutritious as possible. The intent is not to limit your food preparation or eating to any particular list of recipes, but to empower you to apply your new skills as you see fit. Therefore, here are just a few recipes simply to demonstrate how *The Way to Eat* can indeed run right through your kitchen!

Included Recipes

Chewy Granola Squares
Tomato and Red Onion Salad
Sandwich Construction Table
Pasta Dishes

Chewy Granola Squares

These bars provide a very nutritious snack with no added fat that kids love! They are easy and fun to make.

3 cups low-fat granola
1/2 cup chopped hazelnuts
1/2 cup chopped or slivered almonds
1/2 cup chopped walnuts
10 dried figs (the large moist ones!)
1 ripe banana
1/2 cup honey
2 Tbsp. brown sugar
4 egg whites
1/2 cup oat flour
1 cup raw oats
Optional: 1 Tbsp. flaxseeds (freshly ground so they do not lose their nutritional value)

Nutrition Facts	
% of calories per serving	
Serving size: 1 square	

Amount per serving	
Calories 80	Calories from Fat 20

	% Daily Value*
Total Fat 2.5g 4%	28%
Saturated Fat 0g	0%
Polyunsaturated Fat 1g	10%
Monounsaturated Fat 1g	10%
Trans Fat 0g	
Cholesterol 0mg	0%
Sodium 10mg	
Total Carbohydrate 13g 4%	65%
Dietary Fiber 1g	6%
Sugars 7g	35%
Protein 2g	10%

*Percent Daily Values (DV) are based on a 2,000 calorie diet.
Noteworthy Nutrition: provide a variety of nutrients and healthy oils from nuts and seeds

Grind the granola, nuts, and dried fruit together in a food processor until well mixed. Add the rest of the ingredients to the mixture and grind again until the consistency is that of a sticky paste (2 minutes). Place oats in the bottom of an 8x12 pan. Spread the dough with a spatula dipped in water so that it will be easier to handle and finish off the corners with wet fingers, if needed (the kids love to help with this!!!).

Bake in 350 degree oven for 15–20 minutes. Let cool and cut in little squares. Yields 54 squares.

Variation:

Banana bars: Reduce the number of figs to 5 and add 4 dried, whole bananas instead.

Apricot bars: Replace the figs with 14 small dried apricots.

Date bars: Reduce the number of figs to 5 and add 10 dried dates.

Blueberry bars: Reduce the number of figs to 5 and add 1/2 cup dried blueberries.

Cherry bars: Reduce the number of figs to 5 and add 1/2 cup dried cherries.

Tomato and Red Onion Salad

This salad is delicious plain, but is also wonderful used as a basic foundation for other tasty, more complete salads or as a "salsa" over grilled seafood or poultry (see Variations).

Serves 5–6

4 medium ripe but firm tomatoes

1 medium cucumber

1 large red onion

1/2 cup small nicoise olives

1 Tbsp. olive oil

3–4 Tbsp. balsamic vinegar

Pinch of salt and pepper

Chopped basil or cilantro to taste

Nutrition Facts

% of calories per serving
Serving size: 1 small bowl (128g)

Amount per serving	
Calories 35	Calories from Fat 15

	% Daily Value*
Total Fat 1.5g 3%	43%
Saturated Fat 0g	0%
Polyunsaturated Fat 0g	0%
Monounsaturated Fat 1g	26%
Trans Fat 0g	
Cholesterol 0mg	0%
Sodium 50mg	2%
Total Carbohydrate 5g	2%
Dietary Fiber 1g	5%
Sugars 3g	34%
Protein 1g	11%

*Percent Daily Values (DV) are based on a 2,000 calorie diet.

Noteworthy Nutrition: low in calories; rich in vitamin C

1) Peel the cucumber and take out the seeds with a spoon.
2) Dice the cucumbers and tomatoes and slice the red onion finely.
3) Place them in a small salad bowl with the olives.
4) Add the oil, vinegar, salt, and pepper and refrigerate.
5) When ready to serve, top with chopped fresh basil or cilantro to taste.

Variations: Build twelve delicious nutritious salads using the Tomato and Red Onion Salad recipe as a foundation:

1) Add in 2 cups chopped mixed greens.
2) Drizzle one additional teaspoon of olive oil and toss together with either:

- 1 cup cooked fava beans
- 1 clove minced garlic, 1/2 cup crumbled feta, dash of cumin
- 1 cup cooked lentils (mix brown and orange variety), dash of curry
- 1 cup cooked wheat berries, 2 Tbsp. chopped walnuts, dash of turmeric
- 1 cup corn kernels, dash of basil
- 1 cup garbanzo beans, dash of dill
- 1 cup cooked orzo pasta, a sprinkle of fresh grated parmesan (2 Tbsp.)
- 1 cup pearled couscous, 1/2 cup fresh finely chopped mint
- 1 cup fresh asparagus, steamed but crisp and chopped in thirds, 1/2 cup crumbled feta
- 1 cup fresh Brussels sprouts, steamed but not mushy, cut in halves
- 1 fennel bulb, raw, thinly sliced, a dash of fennel seeds
- 1 cup string beans, steamed but crisp, 1/2 chopped hazelnuts
- 1 cup wild rice, 1 1/2 cup diced bell peppers (mix orange, yellow, red, or green for a burst of color)

Any of the Variations above work, with or without the added mixed green or just simply plain, to make the Tomato and Red Onion Salad a salsa or side dish:

Over grilled fish
Over grilled chicken
Over grilled shrimp
Over grilled scallops

Sandwich Construction Table

Choose a bread from column A, your favorite sandwich ingredients from column B, and a nutritious spread from column C. There's plenty here to keep any sandwich enthusiast munching happily, and health-fully, for many lunches to come!

A: Bread	B: Toppings	C: Spreads
Bagel (Whole Grain)	Alfalfa Sprouts	Salsa
	Artichoke Hearts	
Foccacia Bread	Avocado	Chopped Sundried
	Baby Spinach Leaves	Tomatoes
Kaiser Roll	Basil Leaves	
(Whole Grain)	Bean Sprouts	Hummus
	Broccoli Florets	
Olive Bread	(Chopped Raw)	Mustard
	Burger (Salmon)	
	Burger (Tuna)	Olive Tapenade
Onion Bialis	Burger (Veggie)	
	Cabbage (Shredded)	Refried Beans
Pita Bread	Carrots (Shredded)	
(Whole Grain)	Chicken (Grilled Breast)	
	Cucumber	Pureed Roasted
Potato Bread	Eggplant (Grilled)	Red Peppers
	Lettuce	
Sourdough Baguette	Marinated Tofu	Basil Pesto
	Mushroom (Grilled Portabello)	
Tortilla (Corn)	Mushrooms (Sliced Raw)	Cucumber in
	Onions (Caramelized)	Plain Yogurt
Tortilla (Flour)	Onions (Raw)	
	Peppers (Grilled)	Mashed Avocado
Whole-grain Bread (Sliced)	Peppers (Roasted Red in Jar)	Caramelized Onions
	Salmon (Canned Packed in Water)	
Wrap (Whole Grain)	Salmon (Fresh Grilled)	Roasted Garlic
	Tomato (Sliced Raw)	
	Tuna (Canned Packed in Water)	
	Tuna (Fresh Grilled)	
	Turkey (Grilled Skinless Breast)	
	Turkey (Sliced)	
	Zucchini (Grilled)	

Pasta Dishes

Here's a "Chinese menu" approach to many nights of delicious Italian food! Just pick your favorite pastas from column A; sauté, grill, or steam your favorite toppings from column B; and pour over a favorite sauce from column C. Pasta was reportedly invented in the Orient; this approach brings it back home.

A: Pasta	B: Toppings	C: Sauces
Angel Hair	**Vegetables**	Balsamic Vinaigrette
	Artichoke Hearts	
Capellini	Asparagus	
	Bell Peppers	
	Broccoli	Basil Pesto
Cavatelli	Corn	
	Eggplant	
Farfalle	Fennel	Olive Oil & Garlic
	Fresh Tomatoes	
	Leeks	
Fettucine	Mushrooms	Marinara Sauce
	Olives/Capers	
Gnocci	Onions	
	Peas	
	Snow Peas	
Lasagna	Spinach	
	Sundried Tomatoes	
Linguine	Zucchini	
	Seafood	
Macaroni	Clams	
	Crab	
	Lobster	
Orzo	Mussels	
	Salmon (Canned)	
Penne	Scallops	
	Shrimp	

A: Pasta	B: Toppings	C: Sauces
Shells	Squid (Calamari)	
	Tuna (Canned)	
Spaghetti	Salmon (Fresh)	
	Tuna (Fresh)	
Whole-wheat	**Meat**	
	Skinless Chicken	
	Skinless Turkey	
Ziti	Lean Beef	
	Lean Ground Turkey	
	Beans	
	Black Beans	
	Cannelini	
	Fava Beans	
	Garbanzo Beans	
	Green Beans	

Resource 12: *The Way to Find Additional Expert Help*

The Way to Eat is intended to serve as a comprehensive guide as you set out to find and follow a lifetime of good eating habits. The skills and strategies, knowledge and power, provided in the text should prepare you well for the many challenges you will face. But no matter how well prepared you are, sometimes a little expert support is just the thing!

Whether for reinforcing what you already know, troubleshooting a particularly resistant "obstacle," coming up with some new recipe ideas, or enhancing your creativity as you encounter new situations and new challenges, there may be times when you need—or at least want—help. And that help is available. Dietitians can help you overcome any challenge to healthful eating. Well-chosen magazines, newsletters, cook books, software programs, and websites provide useful and current information. If and when the going gets particularly tough, you don't need to be tough all on your own. Get the personalized guidance and support you need from the resources listed below to smooth out any rough spots along your way.

Find a Dietitian

The American Dietetic Association's website, www.eatright.org, offers a national referral service to locate a Registered Dietitian near you.

The National Center for Nutrition and Dietetics (NCND) Information Line is: http://www.eatright.org/ncnd.html.

The Consumer Nutrition Information Line (800-366-1655) offers the public direct access to objective, credible food and nutrition information from the experts—Registered Dietitians. ADA's Consumer Nutrition Information Line provides recorded messages with timely, practical nutrition information as well as referrals to registered dieticians. Messages are available twenty-four hours daily. Messages and accompanying Nutrition Fact Sheets (in English and Spanish) change monthly and offer practical, creative ways to balance food choices for a healthful eating style. Funding for this toll-free service is provided by educational grants to the American Dietetic Association Foundation.

You can contact the ADA headquarters directly by mail or phone:

Headquarters
American Dietetic Association
216 W. Jackson Blvd.
Chicago, IL 60606-6995
(312) 899-0040

Your primary care provider should be able to recommend a dietitian. You may call your local hospital's Nutrition Department and ask to speak to the Outpatient Dietitian. They will generally be happy to help.

In a pinch, the Yellow Pages will probably do! (We're looking into whether finger walking counts toward the recommended thirty minutes of physical activity each day; we'll get back to you…)

Print Resources

Sorting out nutrition fact from fiction as reported in the media can be difficult. Finding reliable sources for accurate nutrition information is essential. The following are our favorites:

Newsletters/Magazines/Articles
Berkeley Wellness Letter
University of California • PO Box 420148
Palm Coast, Florida. 32142 • Telephone: (904) 445-6414
Excellent and credible advice on health promotion,
including nutrition, fitness, and lifestyle

Consumer Reports on Health
Monthly newsletter • Annual subscription price: $24.00
Publisher: Consumers Union of United States, Inc.
101 Truman Avenue • Yonkers, NY 10703-1057
www.consumerreports.org

Environmental Nutrition
Monthly newsletter • Annual subscription price: $30.00
Publisher: Environmental Nutrition, Inc.
52 Riverside Drive, Suite 15-A • New York, NY 10024-6599
www.environmentalnutrition.com

Nutrition Action Health Letter
10 issues a year • Annual subscription price: $24.00
Publisher: The Center for Science in the Public Interest (CSPI)
Suite 300, 1875 Connecticut Avenue, N.W.
Washington, D.C. 20009-5728
Fax: (202) 265-4954 • email: circ@cspinet.org
Consumer advocacy and inside information on commercial
food and nutrition practices with implications for consumer health

Tuft's University Health & Nutrition Letter
Monthly newsletter • Annual subscription price: $28.00
Publisher: Tuft's University
10 High Street, Suite 706 • Boston, MA 02110
www.healthletter.tufts.edu • email: healthletter@tufts.edu
Sound nutrition and health advice from a leading school
of nutrition & medical school

Kostas, G., *Low-fat and Delicious: Can we break the taste barrier?* Journal
of the American Dietetic Association. 1997; 97(supplement): s88-s92.
    *A discussion of methods for translating nutrition guidelines into actual
cooking and eating, available from your area medical library.*

Cookbooks
*(Books listed below are considered particularly helpful, but are a representa-
tive sample only; books to guide nutritious cooking are available by virtually
every category of cuisine and health condition. If you have a specific interest
not addressed below, you should visit an actual or online bookstore.)*
Food Intolerance/Allergy:
Hagman, Bette, *The Gluten-Free Gourmet Cooks Fast and Healthy: Wheat-
    Free with Less Fuss and Fat.* New York: Henry Holt. 1997.
Pannell, Maggie (ed), *Allergy-Free Cooking.* London, England: Lorenz
    Books, 2002.
Diet and Health:
American Heart Association. *American Heart Association Low-Fat, Low-
    Cholesterol Cookbook: Heart-Healthy, Easy-to-Make Recipes That Taste
    Great.* New York: Times Books, 1998.

Castelli, William P., and Griffin, Glen C., *Good Fat, Bad Fat: How to Lower Your Cholesterol and Reduce the Odds of a Heart Attack*. Tucson, AZ: Fisher Books, 1997.

Davis, Brenda, and Vesanto, Melina, *Becoming Vegan: The Complete Guide to Adopting a Healthy Plant-based Diet*. Summertown, TN: Book Publishing Company, 2000.

D'Agostino, Joanne, *Convertible Cooking for a Healthy Heart*. Easton, PA: Hastings House, 1992.

Duyff, Roberta Larson, *The ADA's Complete Food and Nutrition Guide, 2nd Edition*. New York, NY: John Wiley & Sons, 2002.

Editors of the Wellness Cooking School, University of California at Berkeley. *The Wellness Low-fat Cookbook*. New York: Rebus, Inc., 1994.

Editors of the Wellness Cooking School, University of California at Berkeley. *The Simply Healthy Low-fat Cookbook*. New York: Rebus, Inc., 1995.

Lund, Joanne M., and Alpert, Barbara, *Cooking Healthy with the Kids in Mind: A Healthy Exchanges Cookbook*. New York: Perigree, 1998.

Lund, Joanne M., *The Diabetic's Healthy Exchanges Cookbook*. New York: Perigee, 1996.

Vesanto, Melina, and Davis, Brenda, *Becoming Vegetarian: The Complete Guide to Adopting a Healthy Vegetarian Diet*. Summertown, TN: Book Publishing Company, 1995.

Nigro, Shirley, *Companion Guide to Healthy Cooking: A Practical Introduction to Natural Ingredients*. Featherstone, Inc. 1996.

Nixon, Daniel W., et al, *The Cancer Recovery Eating Plan: The Right Foods to Help Fuel Your Recovery*. New York: Times Books, 1996.

Pensiero, Laura, et al, *The Strang Cookbook for Cancer Prevention*. New York: Dutton, 1998.

Ponichtera, Brenda J., *Quick & Healthy Recipes and Ideas: For People Who Say They Don't Have Time to Cook Healthy Meals*. The Dalles, OR: Scaledown, 1991.

Ponichtera, Brenda J., *Quick & Healthy Volume II: More Help for People Who Say They Don't Have Time to Cook Healthy Meals*. The Dulles, OR: Scaledown, 1995.

Rosso, Julee, *Great Good Food*. New York: Crown/Turtle Bay Books, 1993.

Sarubin, Allison, *The Health Professional's Guide to Popular Dietary Suppliments, 2E*. Chicago, IL: American Dietetic Association, 2003.

Shield, Jodie, and Mullen, Mary Catherine, *The ADA Guide to Healthy Eating for Kids*. New York, NY: John Wiley & Sons, 2002.

Starke, Rodman D., and Winston, Mary, (eds), *American Heart Association Low-Salt Cookbook : A Complete Guide to Reducing Sodium and Fat in the Diet*. New York: Times Books, 1990.

Wood, Rebecca, *The New Whole Foods Encyclopedia: A Comprehensive Resource for Healthy Eating*. New York: Penguin Books, 1999.

Other Books of Interest:

Alleman, Gayle Povis, *Save Your Child from the Fat Epidemic*. Rocklin, CA: Prima Publishing, 1999.

Craig, Selene, et al, *The Complete Book of Alternative Nutrition*. Emmaus, PA: Rodale Press, 1997.

Dietz, William H., and Stern, Loraine, (eds), *American Academy of Pediatrics Guide to Your Child's Nutrition*. New York: Villard Books, 1999.

Goodman, Jonathan, *The Omega Solution*. Roseville, CA: Prima Publishing, 2001.

Margen, Sheldon, *The Wellness Nutrition Counter*. New York: Health Letter Associates, 1997.

Murray, Michael T., *Encyclopedia of Nutritional Supplements*. Rocklin, CA: Prima Publishing, 1996.

Neff, Cary, *Conscious Cuisine*. Naperville, IL: Sourcebooks, Inc., 2002.

Rinzler, Carol Ann, *The New Complete Book of Food: A Nutritional, Medical and Culinary Guide*. New York: Checkmark Books, 1999.

Rothfield, Glenn S., et al, *Natural Medicine for Heart Disease*. Emmaus, PA: Rodale Press, 1996.

Somer, Elizabeth, *Food & Mood*. 2nd edition. New York: Henry Holt & Company, 1999.

Tamborlane, William V., (ed), *The Yale Guide to Children's Nutrition*. New Haven, CT: Yale University Press, 1997.

Werbach, Melvin R., *Healing with Food*. New York: HarperPerennial, 1993.

Willett, Walter C., *Eat, Drink and Be Healthy*. New York: Simon & Schuster, 2001.

Web, Software, and Media-based Resource Materials

The following websites are resources for information on nutrition, fitness, and health. Please note that websites come and go; these were up and running when we went to print but we can't guarantee that every one will still be working. Good surfing! (Remember: not too much time at the computer—get in some physical activity!)

Offers a personalized, interactive "Way to Eat" diet planner that includes meal planning, recipe analysis, weight loss guidance, and more, all predicated on the nutrition principles of *The Way to Eat*:

   www.thewaytoeat.net

American Dietetic Association

   www.eatright.org

Webdietitian

   www.webdietitian.com

For personalized online diet, fitness, and motivation programs:

   www.ediets.com

American Heart Association Fitness Center

   www.justmove.org

MayoClinic.com Healthy Lifestyle Planners

   www.mayoclinic.com/home?id=SP6.3.1

The Food Network has a fun website for those who love to cook:

   www.foodtv.com

The U.S. Department of Health and Human Services provides a directory to credible sources of health information on the Web:

   www.healthfinder.gov

These sites allow access to images of the USDA Food Guide Pyramid:

   http://www.nal.usda.gov:8001/py/pmap.htm

   http://www.nalusda.gov/fnic/Fpyr/pyramid.gif

Maintained by the Tufts University School of Nutrition Policy and Science, this site serves as a directory to other nutrition sites for both professional and lay users:

   http://navigator.tufts.edu

On the USDA Nutrient Data Laboratory site, the nutrient composition of virtually any food can be found:

   www.nal.usda.gov/fnic/foodcomp/index.html

This site, maintained by the American Heart Association, provides a wealth of information, including detailed recipes:

   http://www.deliciousdecisions.org

The New York Online Access to Health (NOAH) website provides health information in both English and Spanish:

http://www.noah-health.org/english/wellness/nutrition/nutrition.html

The Personal Nutritionist Website maintained by the American Medical Association allows for individual dietary assessment online, as well as online calculation of BMI from height and weight:

http://www.ama-assn.org/insight/yourhlth/pernutri/pernutri.htm

Essays on topics in health by the U.S. Food and Drug Administration's Center for Food Safety and Applied Nutrition can be found here:

http://vm.cfsan.fda.gov/~dms/wh-nutr.html

This site, maintained by the International Food Information Council, provides consumer-oriented information on food safety:

http://ific.org/food/

This site, maintained by U. S. Food and Drug Administration Center for Food Safety and Applied Nutrition, provides detailed information on the interpretation of food labels, including their use for specific health goals:

http://vm.cfsan.fda.gov/label.html

A private foundation, the Nemours Center for Children's Health Media, maintains this website that offers detailed information on nutrition for the newborn. The site is listed on the healthfinder website. Information on diet and nutrition for older children, through adolescence, is easily accessible from this site:

http://www.kidshealth.org/parent/nutrition_fit/nutrition/feednewborn.html

This site is maintained by the National Center for Diabetes, Digestive, and Kidney Diseases (NIDDK) at the National Institutes of Health, and provides extensive references in the management of diabetes:

http://www.niddk.nih.gov/health/diabetes/pubs/cookbook/cookbook.htm

This site provides a "virtual cookbook" maintained by the Mayo Foundation for Medical Education and Research of the Mayo Clinic. You can select from a variety of recipes, and see the nutritional composition for "standard" and "modified" recipes side by side:

http://www.mayoclinic.com/findinformation/healthylivingcenter

This site, maintained by the National Center for Diabetes, Digestive, and

Kidney Diseases (NIDDK) at the National Institutes of Health provides information on how to avoid weight gain during smoking cessation:

http://www.niddk.nih.gov/health/nutrit/pubs/quitsmok/index.htm

This site is maintained by the National Cancer Institute at the NIH and provides detailed information on diet tailored for patients with cancer:

www.cancer.gov/cancer_information/coping

This site, maintained by the Food and Drug Administration Center for Food Safety and Applied Nutrition, provides information on safe food handling and preparation:

http://www.foodsafety.gov/~fsg/fsgadvic.html

This is the home page for Take Off Pounds Sensibly, an international club providing information and support for sensible weight loss:

http://www.tops.org/

This site, maintained by the National Heart, Lung, and Blood Institute at the NIH, provides guidance in choosing a safe and reasonable weight-loss program:

http://www.nhlbi.nih.gov/health/public/heart/obesity/lose_wt/wtl_prog.htm

This site, maintained by the National Institute of Diabetes, Digestive, and Kidney Diseases at the NIH, provides guidance in choosing a safe and reasonable weight-loss program:

http://www.niddk.nih.gov/health/nutrit/pubs/choose.htm

The nutrition section of WebMD, providing a variety of informative links, is available at:

http://my.webmd.com/nutrition

Selected Federal Resources:

http://www.health.gov/dietaryguidelines/

HHS and USDA provide many sources of information on nutrition and health. Selected resources are listed below.

Healthfinder, HHS's gateway to reliable health information, including diet, nutrition, healthy lifestyle, and physical activity:

www.healthfinder.gov

USDA's gateway to nutrition information:

www.nutrition.gov

FDA's gateway to federal food safety information:
   www.foodsafety.gov
National Action Plan on Overweight and Obesity:
   www.surgeongeneral.gov/topics/obesity
Cancer Information Service, National Cancer Institute, NIH, HHS:
   www.nci.nih.gov/cancer_information
Center for Food Safety and Applied Nutrition, FDA, HHS:
   www.efsan.fda.gov
Centers for Disease Control and Prevention, HHS:
   www.cdc.gov
Center for Nutrition Policy and Promotion, USDA:
   www.usda.gov/cnpp
Food and Nutrition Information Center, National Agricultural Library,
USDA:
   www.nal.usda.gov/fnic
Food and Nutrition Service, USDA:
   www.fns.usda.gov/fns
National Heart, Lung, and Blood Institute, NIH, HHS:
   www.nhlbi.nih.gov
National Institute of Diabetes and Digestive and Kidney Diseases,
NIH, HHS:
   www.niddk.nih.gov
National Institute on Alcohol Abuse and Alcoholism, NIH, HHS:
   www.niaaa.nih.gov

Other Sites of Potential Interest:
   www.nutrio.com
   www.dietquest.com
   www.cyberdiet.com
   www.environmentalnutrition.com

Cable Television:
Food & Nutrition Network
A variety of programs devoted to cooking, nutrition, and the joy of eating. Check area listings.

Bibliography

Primary Source:

Katz, D.L., *Nutrition in Clinical Practice*. Philadelphia, PA: Lippincott Williams & Wilkins, 2000. This text includes citations for some two thousand scientific publications that underlie the views expressed in *The Way to Eat*.

Other Sources of Particular Interest:

American Dietetic Association. Position of the American Dietetic Association: *Food Fortification and Dietary Supplements*. Journal of the American Dietetic Association. 2001; 101:115-125.

American Dietetic Association. Position of the American Dietetic Association: *Health Implications of Dietary Fiber*. Journal of the American Dietetic Association. 1997: 97:1157-1159.

American Dietetic Association. Position of the American Dietetic Association: *The Role of Nutrition in Health Promotion and Disease Prevention Programs*. Journal of the American Dietetic Association. 1998; 98: 205-208.

American Dietetic Association. Position of the American Dietetic Association: *Total Diet Approach to Communicating Food and Nutrition Information*. Journal of the American Dietetic Association. 2002; 102: 100-108.

American Dietetic Association. Position of the American Dietetic Association: *Vegetarian Diets*. Journal of the American Dietetic Association. 1997; 97: 1317-1321.

American Dietetic Association. Position of the American Dietetic Association: *Weight Management*. Journal of the American Dietetic Association. 1997; 97: 71-74.

Boaz, Noel T., and Almquist, Alan J., *Biological Anthropology. A Synthetic Approach to Human Evolution*. Upper Saddle River, NJ: Prentice Hall, 1997.

Eaton, S.B., Eaton, S.B. III, and Konner, M.J., *Paleolithic Nutrition Revisited: A Twelve-Year Retrospective on Its Nature and Implications*. European Journal of Clinical Nutrition. 1997; 51:207-216.

Glanz, K., Basil, M., Maibach, E., Goldberg, J., and Snyder, D., *Why Americans Eat What They Do: Taste, Nutrition, Cost, Convenience, and Weight Control Concerns As Influences on Food Consumption*. Journal of the American Dietetic Association. 1998; 98: 1118-1126.

Institute of Medicine. *Improving America's Diet and Health. From Recommendations to Action*. Washington, D.C.: National Academy Press, 1991.

Neel, J., *Diabetes mellitus: A "Thrifty" Genotype Rendered Detrimental by "Progress"?* American Journal of Human Genetics. 1962; 14: 353-362.

Nestle, M., and Jacobson, M.F., "Halting the Obesity Epidemic: A Public Health Policy Approach." *Public Health Reports*. 2000; 115: 12-24.

Nestle, M., et al, "Behavioral and Social Influences on Food Choice." *Nutritional Review*. 1998; 56 (suppl 2): s50-s74.

Tannahill, Reay, *Food in History*. Upper Saddle, NJ: Three Rivers Press, 1988.

Index

About the Authors

DAVID L. KATZ, M.D., M.P.H., F.A.C.P.M., F.A.C.P. is the nutrition columnist for *O, the Oprah Magazine*, contributing a monthly feature entitled "The Way to Eat." He is the recipient of an award for excellence in health guidance from Healthy U, a nonprofit organization based in Maryland. A board-certified specialist in both Internal and Preventive Medicine, he is Associate Clinical Professor of Public Health & Medicine, and Director of Medical Studies in Public Health, at the Yale University School of Medicine. He co-founded and directs Yale's Prevention Research Center, and founded and directs The Integrative Medicine Center in Derby, CT, where he provides clinical care in a holistic context. He has authored six other books, including *Cut Your Cholesterol* (Reader's Digest, 2004) and a nutrition textbook widely used in medical education (including the Harvard & Yale Medical Schools), and nearly seventy scientific papers. Dr. Katz earned his B.A. from Dartmouth College, his M.D. from the Albert Einstein College of Medicine, and his MPH from the Yale School of Medicine.

Dr. Katz lectures on nutrition, health promotion, and disease prevention throughout the U.S. and abroad. In 2003, he was a featured speaker on the topic of weight control at the "Steps to a Healthier U.S. Summit" convened by the U.S. Secretary of Health, and a keynote speaker at both Canada's Healthy Living Symposium, convened by the Ministry of Health, and the Canadian Cardiovascular Congress. His expert opinion has been featured on ABC's "20/20", PBS, Fox News, WebMD, the BBC, and Canada's "Balance" television program. In October 2003, he was featured in a *TIME* magazine cover story on "eating smart." His expert opinion is regularly cited in *O, The Oprah Magazine, Good Housekeeping, Prevention, Glamour, Shape, Child, Self, Men's Health, Muscle & Fitness,* as well as the *New York Times, Washington Post, Boston Globe, Wall Street Journal,* and many others. Dr. Katz has been called on by the U.S. Secretary of Health, the Commissioner of the Food & Drug Administration, and an obesity control task force convened by the Governor of Florida, to provide expert recommendations for obesity prevention and control.

Dr. Katz lives in Connecticut with his wife, Catherine, and their five children: Rebecca, Corinda, Valerie, Natalia, and Gabriel.

MAURA HARRIGAN GONZÁLEZ, M.S., R.D. is a Registered Dietitian with over twenty years of clinical nutrition experience in hospital and private practice settings. She formerly served as the Research Dietitian at the Yale Prevention Research Center and maintains a private practice in nutrition counseling. González earned her bachelor's degree in Food and Nutrition from the University of North Carolina. She completed her Dietetic Internship at the New York Hospital-Cornell Medical Center and obtained her master's degree in Clinical Nutrition from New York University. González is certified in Adult Weight Management by the American Dietetic Association.

González was formerly the head dietitian at the Payne Whitney Psychiatric Clinic of the New York Hospital. She then served as Chief Clinical Dietitian, and subsequently Associate Director of Nutrition at Saint Vincent's Medical Center in New York City. She was awarded the Recognized Young Dietitian Award from the American Dietetic Association.

González lives in Connecticut with her husband, Carlos, a psychiatrist, and their two daughters, Gabriela and Ana. Active in local politics, González serves as an elected member of the Board of Education where she advocates the integration of nutrition education and healthy lifestyles into the curriculum at the elementary school level. Come every spring, you'll find her out on the softball field coaching her daughters' team, the Rockies.